Preparing the Perfect Medical CV

A comprehensive guide for doctors and medical students on how to succeed in your chosen field

Second Edition

Helen Douglas & Vivek Sivarajan
Edited by Matt Green

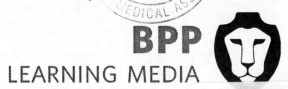

BPP
LEARNING MEDIA

First edition 2010
Second edition September 2011

ISBN 9781 4453 8162 6
Previous ISBN 9780 9556 7463 1
e-ISBN 9781 4453 8587 7

British Library Cataloguing-in-Publication Data
A catalogue record for this book is available
from the British Library

Published by
BPP Learning Media Ltd
BPP House, Aldine Place
London W12 8AA

www.bpp.com/health

Typeset by Replika Press Pvt Ltd, India
Printed in the United Kingdom

Your learning materials, published by BPP
Learning Media Ltd, are printed on paper
sourced from sustainable, managed forests.

The views expressed in this book are those of
BPP Learning Media and not those of the NHS.
BPP Learning Media are in no way associated
with or endorsed by the NHS.

The contents of this book are intended as a guide
and not professional advice. Although every effort
has been made to ensure that the contents of
this book are correct at the time of going to
press, BPP Learning Media, the Editor and the
Author make no warranty that the information
in this book is accurate or complete and accept
no liability for any loss or damage suffered by
any person acting or refraining from acting as
a result of the material in this book.

Every effort has been made to contact the
copyright holders of any material reproduced
within this publication. If any have been
inadvertently overlooked, BPP Learning Media
will be pleased to make the appropriate credits
in any subsequent reprints or editions.

A note about copyright

Dear Customer

What does the little © mean and why
does it matter?

Your market-leading BPP books, course
materials and e-learning materials
do not write and update themselves.
People write them on their own behalf
or as employees of an organisation
that invests in this activity. Copyright
law protects their livelihoods. It does
so by creating rights over the use of
the content.

Breach of copyright is a form of theft
– as well as being a criminal offence
in some jurisdictions, it is potentially a
serious beach of professional ethics.

With current technology, things might
seem a bit hazy but, basically, without
the express permission of BPP Learning
Media:

• Photocopying our materials is a
  breach of copyright
• Scanning, ripcasting or conversion
  of our digital materials into different
  file formats, uploading them to
  facebook or e-mailing them to your
  friends is a breach of copyright

You can, of course, sell your books, in
the form in which you have bought them
– once you have finished with them.
(Is this fair to your fellow students?
We update for a reason.)   But the
e-products are sold on a single user
license basis: we do not supply 'unlock'
codes to people who have bought them
secondhand.

And what about outside the UK?
BPP Learning Media strives to make
our materials available at prices
students can afford by local printing
arrangements, pricing policies and
partnerships which are clearly listed
on our website. A tiny minority ignore
this and indulge in criminal activity by
illegally photocopying our material or
supporting organisations that do. If they
act illegally and unethically in one area,
can you really trust them?

ii

BPP
LEARNING MEDIA

Contents

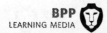

Section 2: Application forms

Section 3: Portfolio structure

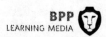

About the Publisher

BPP Learning Media is dedicated to supporting aspiring professionals with top quality learning material. BPP Learning Media's commitment to success is shown by our record of quality, innovation and market leadership in paper-based and e-learning materials. BPP Learning Media's study materials are written by professionally-qualified specialists who know from personal experience the importance of top quality materials for success.

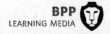

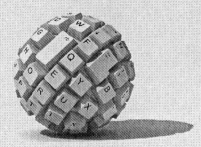

Free Companion Material

Readers can access a template CV in Word, which they can adapt, for free online.

To access the above companion material please visit **www.bpp.com/freehealthresources**

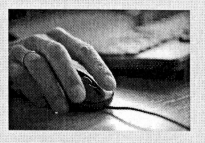

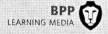

About the Authors

Helen Douglas

Helen is a graduate of Sheffield Medical School. She completed her PRHO year in General and Paediatric Medicine and Surgery, her F2 year in Anatomy Demonstrating and A&E, and her Specialist Training in Plastic Surgery, completing rotations in Plastics, ENT, Orthopaedics and General Surgery. She spent the last two years as the Laser Research Fellow at Canniesburn Plastic Surgery Unit in Glasgow, reading for on MD. She has recently commenced a run-through training post at ST3 level in Plastic Surgery in Yorkshire.

Vivek Sivarajan

Vivek is a Consultant Plastic Surgeon, one of the youngest of his generation. Vivek has had a flawless medical career and now participates in trainee recruitment and appraisal. Vivek has a clear understanding of what is required to succeed in every stage of your medical career.

About the Editor

Matt Green

Matt has been assisting doctors of all grades and specialties to improve their CVs for a number of years. It is with this in mind that he has edited this book to pass on his wisdom in this field.

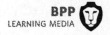

Acknowledgements

We would like to acknowledge with gratitude the help and support of the following people, without whom the writing of this guide would have been difficult if not impossible.

Dr John Bache (Retired Consultant in A&E Medicine, Leighton)

Mr Christopher West (Specialist Registrar in Plastic Surgery, Edinburgh)

Miss Sarah Chadwick (Research Fellow in Plastic Surgery, Manchester)

Mr James Tiernan (Specialist Registrar in General Surgery, Sheffield)

Helen Douglas & Vivek Sivarajan

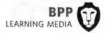

Foreword

Progressing your medical career is a challenging but ultimately rewarding experience that few other vocations offer. Regardless of the stage you are at, the sooner you take a proactive approach to developing and matching your skills and experience to your intended career path, the better. Whether you are a medical student looking to successfully apply to the Foundation Programme or an accomplished Consultant looking to gain acceptance on to a specialist committee, you must always be clear on what those evaluating your application will be looking for.

The main aim of this guide is to tell you, the reader, exactly how to present your CV or application form in a manner that will help you to stand out over your rival applicants. It also provides readers with a clear insight into what steps you should take to develop your skills and how to gain involvement in activities that will benefit you and your career in the long-term. It may be an old adage, but 'Success comes to those who prepare for it!'

It may be the case that you have purchased this book with simply applying to one post in mind. However, the goal of publishing this book is to support individuals in their job applications at every step of their career.

The process of applying for a new post is daunting, and something that we have all experienced at one stage or another. Consequently, it has given me great pleasure in distilling the experience I have gained over the years into this guide.

Remember, a poorly structured and presented CV can let down even those with the most illustrious of careers! Please take the time to fully absorb the contents to avoid the common mistakes and pitfalls that many individuals make, and in doing so stand out for the right reasons.

On that note, may I wish you the best of luck with your current and future applications!

Matt Green

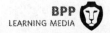

Introduction

Whether you are thinking of applying to Medical School, finishing your Foundation 1 year, choosing your future specialty or completing your training, the competition to secure your next position is overwhelming at every stage and always has been. However, the current climate of UK medical training, particularly in light of the problems with the Medical Training and Applications System (MTAS) and the uncertain future regarding MMC, means that the application process is more frequent, more challenging and different every year. The competition for training posts is incredibly steep, as the government workforce planning for medical staff has made no secret of the fact that despite decreasing referral-to-treatment times to eighteen weeks, doctors' training numbers are being cut. The result? Massive increase in competition for training numbers and rock-bottom morale amongst the medical community. Never has it been so important to be able to present yourself as a suitable candidate for jobs, and it is easy to become despondent when considering the extent of competition. However, it is important to remember that these positions are out there and available, and by presenting yourself in the best possible light you will gain the highest chance of securing the place you want.

This guide is not a magic wand. It will not transform your experiences and qualifications into those needed for a place at Medical School, or a particular job or fellowship. However, it will help you to identify steps that you can take at various stages before your applications to achieve extra material for your CV and help you to display concisely the evidence you have to those selecting candidates. We make some points, particularly concerning CV construction, in more than one chapter. Because of that, when considering an application you can safely refer to the chapter that specifically relates to your level of training, whilst keeping in mind the preparation points that are relevant for the next stage of training. Tending to your CV is a constant process; every job, course and experience you complete will add

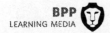

vital evidence of your suitability and eligibility for a position. Therefore it is wise to start preparing for the next job you want as soon as you have secured your current position. This may sound exhausting, and at times never-ending, but as a medic you have by nature an enquiring scientific mind, perform well under pressure and have skills in organisation. It is far easier to justify an application to a particular specialty if you have shown evidence of gaining insight and experience into that field.

Try to set aside some time twice a year (preferably not the day before your annual review meeting) to do a little CV nurturing. Add in the skills/courses/exam results you have achieved over the past six months, update your address and contact numbers if relevant and minister to your career intentions. Keep a copy of your CV saved in your email account, either in the storage facility or sent to yourself as an email. This way wherever you are, even if you are abroad on elective or fellowship, you can keep it updated like a log-book and are unlikely to forget or overlook items to add, which is all too easy to do if you only update it once a year.

Above all, remember that medicine is a vocation, a career, a science and an art. Achieving your desired post is indeed a worthy cause of celebration, and hard work towards that goal is justified. However, it is not worth becoming unwell in your pursuit of it. If you are feeling overwhelmed or unable to cope at any stage, do not suffer in silence. Talk to your friends, colleagues, seniors, GP or Occupational Health Department early. Many of them will have been through the same stresses and may be able to help you simply by sharing their experiences.

Good luck to you all and if you find yourself questioning why you are doing all of this for the pursuit of a job, I would like to quote to you my first ever Mentor and Consultant in Sheffield, the inimitable Consultant General and Transplant Surgeon, Mr Andrew Raftery. 'Are you happy in your work, Ma'am?' My answer was invariably yes. I wish you all happiness in your work also.

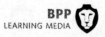

Chapter 1

Covering letters

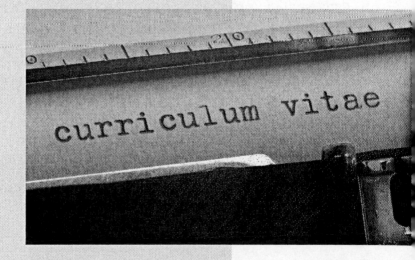

Covering letters

At this point, you may be asking why a chapter has been set aside to include covering letters, when training applications are usually done online and CVs are brought to interview or emailed to the shortlisters. Whilst this is true, when applying for some jobs it is still advisable to submit a covering letter too. If you are not one of the lucky few who enjoy a seamless run-through training opportunity, you may well think of enhancing your CV with a Research Fellow position, which will improve your research skills and help you learn to produce good quality publications and presentations; or a Clinical Fellow post, to increase your clinical experience at a particular level. These posts, usually advertised through NHS Jobs or BMJ Careers, require the applicant to submit in several ways according to the deanery advertising. If they ask you to submit a CV as part of the application process, it is usually wise to include a covering letter, unless specifically instructed not to. The inclusion of such a letter is traditional and makes your application look professional and mature.

Covering letters can be adapted for any level, and follow a very simple and similar format, therefore there is no need to tailor yours to any specific level of training. Instead just keep it up to date as your career progresses. The covering letter should include your contact details and a short description of your current position, relevant experience and qualifications for the position (check the person specification very carefully for this.) Below are three examples that could be used for different types of applications.

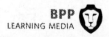

Example covering letter for Associate Specialist application

1 Birch Drive
London
SW1 1AA
Tel: 0207 222 5555
Mob: 07777333000
jjsmith@gmail.com

9 February 2011

Mrs Jane Jones
HR Manager (Senior Medical Staff)
Clinical Excellence
Education Centre
Wirral University Teaching Hospital NHS Foundation Trust

Dear Mrs Jones,

Having recently achieved my Colposcopy and Pelvic Ultrasound Scanning accreditations, as well as having gained my MRCOG, I wish to be considered for the position of Associate Specialist at Wirral University Teaching Hospital.

As you will see from my enclosed curriculum vitae I am currently working as a Trust Doctor in Obstetrics and Gynaecology and am keen to develop skills in colposcopy, gynaecological ultrasound and infertility as sub-specialist interests within the Associate Specialist role.

I would welcome the opportunity to come for interview and can be contacted by telephone, email or letter.

Yours sincerely,

Mr John Smith
MBChB MRCOG
Trust Doctor in Obstetrics & Gynaecology

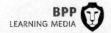

Example covering letter for ENT Research Fellow application

1 Birch Drive
London
SW1 1AA
Tel: 0207 222 5555
Mob: 07777333000
jjsmith@gmail.com

9 February 2011

Mrs Jane Jones
HR Manager (Senior Medical Staff)
Clinical Excellence
Education Centre
Manchester University Teaching Hospital NHS Foundation Trust

Dear Mrs Jones,

Having recently achieved my Membership of the Royal College of Surgeons and having a keen interest in research, I wish to be considered for the position of Research Fellow in Ear Nose and Throat Surgery at Manchester University Teaching Hospital.

As you will see from my enclosed curriculum vitae I am currently working in a Fixed Term Specialty Training appointment post, Year 2, in Ear Nose and Throat Surgery and am keen to develop skills in research whilst maintaining and enhancing my clinical competencies within the Research Fellow role.

I would welcome the opportunity to come for interview and can be contacted by telephone, email or letter.

Yours sincerely,

Mr John Smith
MBChB MRCS
FTSTA SHO in Ear Nose and Throat Surgery

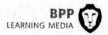

Example covering letter for salaried GP application

> 1 Birch Drive
> London
> SW1 1AA
> Tel: 0207 222 5555
> Mob: 07777333000
> jjsmith@gmail.com
>
> 9 February 2011

Dr J Jones
Willow Surgery
Oak Road
Bristol
BS1 1AA

Dear Dr Jones,

Having gained my MRCGP and recently completed my Diploma in Sexual and Reproductive Health I believe that I am an ideal candidate to be considered for the position of salaried GP which was advertised in BMJ Careers on 12th January.

As you will see from my enclosed curriculum vitae I am currently undertaking locum general practitioner and out-of-hours service cover, and am keen to develop skills in chronic disease management as a special interest within the general practitioner role.

I would welcome the opportunity to come for interview and can be contacted by telephone, email or letter.

Yours sincerely,

Dr John Smith
MBChB MRCGP

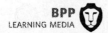

Chapter 2

Application to Medical School

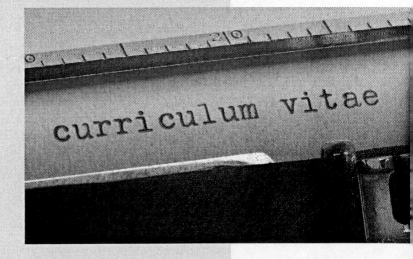

Application to Medical School

Introduction

If you are reading this chapter, then you are considering or have already begun applying for Medical School. In doing so, I am confident that you will already have done sufficient research on the application process and the steps involved. I am also confident that you realise you are embarking on a journey that is long and hard, and may be emotionally, physically and financially challenging. If you are successful in your application and training, this will change your life significantly, as medicine is a vocation and often a lifestyle, not simply a job. The path to becoming a doctor may at times seem frustrating, tiring and endless, however the rewards of an interesting and challenging medical career are abundant.

Why is this book significant to you at this stage of your career? You are not required to submit a CV for Medical School applications, as the Universities and Colleges Admissions Service (UCAS) form requires only a personal statement and references. However, writing a CV that is relevant to your Medical School application is a good idea, because it will give you ideas for your UCAS form, which is split into sections entitled Personal Details, Education, Employment, Additional Information, Personal Statement and References. These can largely be reproduced from the relevant areas of your CV. Also, a well constructed CV will be required if you are applying for placements or jobs related to work experience for Medical School; and if you gain entry to Medical School, you will need a medically oriented CV for the rest of your working life. It will then need constant updating and attention. Therefore there is no better time to start to prepare your medical CV than the present.

The demographic of Medical School applicants has changed significantly in the last few decades, with far more mature students entering medical training than ever before, making 10

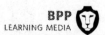

to 15% of Medical School intakes per year. Those of you who are mature students, or are applying after a 'gap' year, will probably already have a CV based on your previous careers and experiences, which you will be able to adapt in light of your new career choice. For others of you at school or college, this application may be the first you have ever made. Regardless of your previous experience, it is important to be able to display a keen enthusiasm for and understanding of medical training and the paths to which it will lead.

As I am sure you know, the competition to enter Medical School is daunting, with many more applicants than spaces available. By being eligible to apply for Medical School, you were all probably the highest academic achievers at school or college. At this stage however, practically all of the applicants for Medical School will be the highest achievers at their own schools or colleges from all over the UK and abroad. Hence, the difficulty for applicants is how to 'stand out' from this tremendously high-calibre crowd, of whom the large majority will look very similar on paper. Unfortunately, with the recent trend for more generically styled application forms and structured standardised interviews, this difficulty will probably continue to present itself in all your future applications. The aim, therefore, is to construct your CV in such a way as to present required and relevant information in the clearest and most coherent way. The material that you have available to put on your CV, and indeed your UCAS form, is the result of the hard work you have already done. Below is a 'Preparation' section, which you can use to check that you have made best use of the evidence of that hard work to increase your chances of securing a place at Medical School.

Ask yourself, 'What are the shortlisters looking for in a Medical School applicant?' The answer is very simple. They are looking for someone who will be able to cope with the academic, personal and emotional pressure of four, five or six years at Medical School, and then be able to make the transition to junior doctor successfully. They are trying to pick the candidates who in the short term will not drop out of or fail Medical School, but also

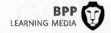

those who already possess the desirable characteristics of a doctor.

Some better-known examples of these characteristics include academic ability; an enquiring mind; the ability to deal well with pressure and make decisions; leadership and teamwork qualities; and enthusiasm and aptitude for teaching. Qualities that are often forgotten, or mistakenly left out as 'soft,' are good communication skills, empathy for other people, honesty, trustworthiness and reliability. If you wish to read more about the qualities, duties and standards of a doctor, go to the General Medical Council website (www.gmc-uk.org) and read a document called *Good Medical Practice*. This document outlines the standards against which all of you who are successful in your quest to become a doctor will measure your practice. Most of these skills will be developed and honed over your years at Medical School, but it is the potential for them that the Medical School applications team are looking to see.

I am a firm believer that you do not have to be excessively clever to get into and get through Medical School. You *do* have to be hardworking, organised and tenacious. You *do* have to like people, be able to empathise with patients and have a desire to help them in all aspects of their healthcare. You *do* have to believe in yourself. And it really helps to have a good support network around you, be that in the form of spouse, parents, siblings or friends. If you can do all of these things, you will not have a problem completing your medical training. All you have to do now is to display to the medical school selection panel why you will be an excellent medical student and even better doctor.

Preparation

As a Medical School applicant, you must show to the applications team that you understand what will be required of you as a medical student and have taken steps to gain experience and knowledge of the medical field.

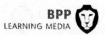

For most of you, this will be the accumulation of many years of hard work and preparation to possess the qualifications and experience to be eligible to apply. If you already have a CV, print it out and examine it critically. Is this the summary of a competitive Medical School applicant? If not, then why not? If you have any medical contacts, then approach them and ask if they would mind having a look at your CV to see if there are any areas where you could improve. Below are areas to concentrate on as early as possible before the applications commence to give yourself the best chance of obtaining a place at Medical School.

Qualifications

The qualifications you will require to get into Medical School vary depending on whether you are an A level student, mature applicant or currently reading another degree. The qualifications required also vary between Medical Schools, and the details are available on each Medical School's website – if there are any issues which are unclear, contact the Medical School undergraduate Admissions Tutor for clarification.

At the time of writing, most Medical Schools require A level grades of AAB, one of which must be Chemistry, and some also require Biology. (Equivalent requirements for Scottish Highers or International Baccalaureate are also available on the medical school websites). Mature students are either expected to achieve these A level grades too, or have a first or upper second-class honours degree in a subject that may or may not need to be related to science. For your application to be successful, you must either already have these academic requirements or be predicted to attain them before the start of Medical School. Therefore please be realistic, as there is no point in spending lots of time and effort applying if you are not going to have the grades required for entry. If you think it is likely that you are not going to be predicted to attain the grades you need, firstly ask yourself why, and be honest about whether or not you can do this. If you are at school or college and you have time to rectify the situation

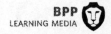

by pulling up your coursework grades, speak to your teachers or tutors and ask honestly what evidence or coursework grades they would require before the applications are due to make them believe that you would attain the required grades. They may need you to put in extra effort out-of-hours or re-take modules, but if you do not ask, you will not know.

If you are a mature student, or did not get the grades you wanted the first time around, you can either re-take these examinations through a local college, or consider applying for foundation courses, which take place in a preliminary year before the start of medical training, where the student has to master the basics required for Biology and Chemistry. Be aware however, that these places are limited and it is hard work to cover what are essentially two A levels in one year.

Work experience

As it is likely that every applicant to Medical School will be predicted the required academic qualifications or indeed already have them, it is vital for you to obtain as many relevant forms of work experience as you can before the application. Organising and completing work experience shows that you have made an effort to work in a caring role, gain experience of a team-related environment and get a feel for how the NHS or its allied organisations work. The school-organised work experience placements that you may have completed are not sufficient; you need to show serious commitment to your Medical School application by putting in extra time, doing extra work to gain extra experience and knowledge that will help you in your future career and show the applications team that you are totally committed to becoming a doctor. This work experience can be paid or voluntary but should be of a decent time period and in a real healthcare environment. Short-duration jobs that may be public-spirited but do not really focus on healthcare, like a week making tea at a warden-sheltered housing association, will not be enough. Common places to try to get experience are nursing homes, community housing or social projects for people with

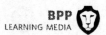

physical or learning difficulties, or hospices. Ideally you need a period of time in these supportive and caring team roles, and then some formal medical shadowing experience, to show that you have addressed several areas of work experience in your spare time. Contact your local hospital or GP surgery and explain that you are trying to acquire some voluntary work experience and would like to shadow some junior doctors in whichever specialty you are most interested in. Yes, all of this is incredibly time-consuming, particularly if you are studying for exams or holding down a full-time job. However, this is the surest way to strengthen your application and I am sure you will find the experiences very rewarding.

Medical career events

There are many events or courses available for potential Medical School applicants, which can be easily found on the Internet or by contacting your school careers advisor or local careers advisory service. These courses aim to give applicants insight into medical training and future career options and information. They often have advice regarding ways to make yourself more competitive for application also. These do provide useful insight, but they are not free of charge and many exist, so if you are interested in these then do some research before booking to make sure you select the course that is appropriate for you.

Teaching

Development of the attitudes, qualities and skills of a teacher is one of the pillars of *Good Medical Practice*, a document mentioned earlier in this chapter. Evidence of enthusiasm for and experience of teaching are desirable qualities in a doctor and can only strengthen your application. Some of you will already have backgrounds that involved teaching, which will strengthen this area of your application, though many of you will not. If you have time before the applications are due, volunteer an afternoon a week of your time to help as an assistant teacher at your previous secondary school, perhaps in

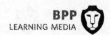

science which would be most relevant. If you are planning to defer to undertake a gap year abroad, perhaps see if you can tailor your plans to involve yourself in teaching at some point. There are plenty of organisations based all over the world that are keen to have volunteer teachers for variable periods of time. Some of these require you to take a course in Teaching English as a Foreign Language (TEFL) but this is a short course which can be taken over a weekend or even online, and could be an extra qualification for your CV! More information on gap year projects and TEFL courses is available online or at any careers advisory service.

Leadership/management

Evidence of leadership ability is advantageous when applying for Medical School, because as a doctor you will be expected to participate in, co-ordinate and lead multidisciplinary teams. Some of you will already have experience of this either in your previous fields of work or in the forms of sporting captaincy or prefect duties etc. If there is a lack of leadership experience on your CV, think if there are any opportunities for you to step up in any organisations or teams you are currently involved in at school, work, sporting or other clubs. Consider if there are any societies or award schemes you could join such as the Duke of Edinburgh award, though these take time and commitment, and if there is less than a year before your applications are due in you are unlikely to be able to show completion. However, evidence of participation could be recorded on your CV/UCAS form. If you have a free summer before the applications it may be worthwhile applying for some form of volunteer or paid summer camp experience, at home or abroad, where you may be leading, teaching or organising sporting events for children or adolescents.

Interests/extra-curricular activities

If you are already involved in many extra-curricular activities that display you as a good all-rounder, then very little preparation is

14

needed for this section. If not, then think realistically about what you can achieve in terms of this section as well as studying for your exams and doing work experience. If there is a particular hobby you have always wanted to try then perhaps give it a go; consider joining school/college activities or societies, but only if you are interested in them. Your local community centre will have lots of information on evening classes and courses, and if you are interested in trying them they may end up as a talking-point on your CV and at interview. Other organisations that you may consider joining could include local charity or volunteering services. Perhaps pick a charity that appeals to you individually. This could also serve to show leadership potential if you are given a role of responsibility.

 ## Key preparation points

- Prepare early
- Assess your likely predicted grades early, and if these are not up to standard, take steps to try to improve them
- Apply for work experience early and to more than one place/ environment, ie nursing home and local hospital department
- Consider attending a medical careers event
- Consider volunteering as an assistant teacher or tailoring your gap year to include teaching
- Consider applying for leadership-style roles such as camp leader, or official in school or college societies
- Consider taking up more extra-curricular activities or classes
- Consider volunteering for a local charity

 ## Key CV construction points

- Always put everything in reverse chronological order (most recent first). The most recent things you have done are of most interest to the applications team
- Avoid fancy fonts: ease of reading is the aim! Arial, Calibri, Cambria are personal favourites, but any font which is clear and easy to read is unlikely to offend
- Font size – keep it size ten or above, twelve if possible. A shortlister that is reading dozens of CVs is likely to be irritated if they need to squint

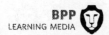

- Paragraphs: to save space, do not start a new paragraph unnecessarily
- Spacing: you will extend the length of the CV if you double-space everything
- 'I': avoid the use of the word 'I' as it can become very repetitive
- Length: historically the 'keep to two pages' rule has been applied. We would recommend less than five and more than one
- Alignment: try to keep everything symmetrical and in alignment. There are fancy computer programs that can do this for you, but a keen eye, printing out a test copy and looking at it carefully will do the same job
- Bold and underlining: avoid overuse. Employ headings to highlight areas of importance and use the bold function sparingly. Do not be tempted to mix and match these throughout the CV, as it will cause confusion. Stick to one
- Bullets: can be very useful to list items succinctly but do not overuse them

Writing the CV

Personal/professional details

Include your full name, address and telephone contacts, and a sensible-sounding email address.

Qualifications and prizes/distinctions

If you already have a degree, always include the university or professional body that awarded it, the inclusive dates and a short summary of the course or subject. List your actual or predicted A level grades along with your GCSE qualifications.

Employment

If you are applying as a mature student then list any relevant previous employment here, particularly if it relates to medicine, eg nursing or support work. Any paid work experience in medically allied fields should also be listed here, in reverse chronological order as always. As job titles are often vague and do not reflect the full capacity of a particular role, include a short summary

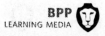

of your roles and responsibilities in this position, so that the shortlisters can see your previous experience and skills.

Courses

If you are applying from a medically related background then you may already have completed some courses involving skills such as resuscitation, ECGs or phlebotomy. List courses with their dates (in reverse chronological order as always) and also the location and professional body involved, eg the Resuscitation Council for BLS. Include courses such as Teaching English as a Foreign Language, management courses and any other non-medical courses which relate to the headings on your CV.

Teaching

If you have any formal teaching experience, then list it here with an explanation of your title and role, the target ages and levels of the people you were teaching, the dates the teaching was delivered over and a brief summary of what it involved. You may wish to include a short statement regarding your awareness of the importance of teaching skills and ability relevant to the medical field. For example:

> I have always been interested in teaching others, and feel this is a vital part of a doctor's duty to more junior trainees. My teaching experience includes six months' formal teaching as a classroom assistant and gap year experience teaching English as a foreign language for six months.

Leadership/management

Any positions that you have held where you were responsible for other people or teams should be listed here with a brief explanation. For example, say if you have captained any sports, led any organisations or held any jobs which involved team leading or positions of responsibility. Again, a brief statement highlighting your awareness of the importance of leadership

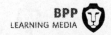

and management qualities for a doctor could be useful before listing your experience. For example:

> I recognise the need for a medical student and indeed doctor to possess good teamworking, leadership and management skills to function effectively in such a multidisciplinary field. My experience in this area includes:
>
> - Two years as Hampshire County Netball Captain
> - Three years experience as a bar manager in a large chain restaurant, organising a team of staff

Interests

Use this section to display yourself as a good all-rounder, who enjoys many activities outside of school. Sports, music, theatre, dance – all are relevant. If you have any prizes or awards in these interests such as musical grades or martial art grading levels, then list them here.

Career intentions/why medicine

A summary statement regarding your career intentions should be included here but should be brief and succinct. This statement needs to address three areas:

- Why you wish to pursue a career in medicine
- What efforts you have made to increase your insight and experience
- What qualities you possess to make you a suitable medical student

Avoid any statements which suggest that you are 'set' on any particular medical specialty yet, as this will look unrealistic and immature – you have not yet started medical training, therefore how can you know with any informed certainty that you want to be an Ear, Nose and Throat surgeon? You can however, make a

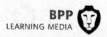

brief statement regarding your interest in a particular specialty if you can back this up with some work experience. Explaining why you want to do medicine is sometimes more difficult than it seems. Feel free to draw from personal experiences but avoid overly dramatic or nostalgic statements. For example, an appropriate statement might be: 'I have wanted to pursue medicine as a career since breaking my leg as a child and respecting the knowledge, empathy and teamwork of the medical staff involved with my care' rather than' I have dreamed of being a doctor since I was four years old, having had a near-fatal car crash and being saved by the heroic efforts of the senior doctor'.

As well as personal experiences, an objective assessment of why you want to do medicine is probably beneficial also. This often involves the rolling-out of the old 'I love people and I love science' statement, which is often ridiculed by medical students (only after they have secured their place at Medical School using such a statement of course). But however cheesy it might sound, if it is true and you really are a sociable science-lover, then try to be more specific about what makes you feel that way and word it to reflect your own genuine opinions. A summary of the qualities that you possess that you feel would make you suitable as a medical student would be a good closing statement. Avoid a long list as this risks making you seem arrogant. For example:

I have been interested in pursuing a career in medicine since beginning secondary school, after a talk from junior and senior doctors at a careers awareness day. As a keen science student I have always wanted to combine my interest in biology and chemistry with a career that allows me to interact and communicate effectively with people, and I feel that medicine is such a science and art. I understand that medicine is a competitive and demanding career and have striven to increase my insight into my chosen field by talking to medical students and doctors, performing work experience at local hospitals and securing a job in a healthcare-related field. I am particularly drawn to paediatrics, but am keen to experience all community and hospital specialties. I am predicted the requisite A level results

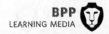

for Medical School entry and feel certain I can achieve these. I believe that I have the qualities required for a good medical student; I am hard working, organised, diligent and focused and feel that I would perform well at Medical School.

Referees

If you are applying straight from school, then your teachers will be your referees. Usually this will be a science teacher or head teacher that knows you well. If you are a mature applicant, your previous employer or perhaps further educational supervisor may be people to ask for a reference.

Approach them early and in person, and ask if they would be willing to support your application to Medical School. Offer them a copy of your CV, detailing your work experience and extra-curricular activities, so that they may draw from this when writing their reference, and try to give them an idea of the application schedule so that they can prepare it at the right time. Ensure they have it done before going to a conference or away on holiday.

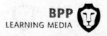

Example CV for application to Medical School

John James Smith

Date of birth:	1 January 1991
Nationality:	British
Address:	1 Birch Drive, London SW1 1AA
Telephone:	0207 222 5555/0777333000
E-mail:	jjsmith@gmail.com

QUALIFICATIONS

2007–Present	**St Sixth Form College, London**	**Predicted A level grades**
Mathematics		A
Biology		A
Chemistry		A
Spanish		B
General Studies		A

2002–2007	**St Secondary School, London**	**GCSE grades**
English Language		A*
English Literature		A
Mathematics		A*
Biology		A*
Chemistry		A
Physics		A
French		A
German		A
Geography		A*
Music		B

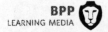

EMPLOYMENT

Aug 2008–Present   Health Care Assistant, London NHS Trust

I am currently working part-time during weekends and holidays at a community-based house that provides support for adults with physical and learning disabilities. I am involved in all aspects of daily care for the clients including support with personal and social activities. This position has improved my teamworking and responsibility skills; I enjoy this work immensely and feel it has provided me with valuable insight into a healthcare environment.

Jun 08–Aug 08   Activity Leader, Camp Castaway, Alabama, USA

During my summer holidays I spent ten weeks working for Camp Castaway, as an Activity leader. I was responsible for a dormitory of campers aged 8–12. I organised and led social and sporting activities, supported by senior staff. This position improved my leadership and teaching skills and enhanced my independence and creativity.

Aug 06–June 07   Waiter, Harvester Restaurant, London

As a college student I worked as a waiter at a busy chain restaurant in London. This job helped to develop my organisation and teamworking skills.

WORK EXPERIENCE

Aug 08–Present   Health Care Assistant, London NHS Trust

Please see above summary.

Nov 07   Paediatric Department, Local Hospital, London

As part of my school Work Experience Programme, I spent two weeks shadowing doctors in the paediatric department of my local hospital. I attended ward rounds, clinics and multi-disciplinary team meetings, and observed the junior and senior medical staff in their day-to-day work. This experience gave me valuable insight into hospital-based paediatric medicine and the types of roles, some of the conditions and pathologies treated and the roles within the health care team.

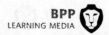

TEACHING

I have always been interested in teaching others, and feel this is a vital part of a doctor's duty to more junior trainees. During the past year I have spent one afternoon a week volunteering as a classroom assistant at my old secondary school, helping to teach science to Year 7 students. I have gained valuable teaching experience during this time and helped to teach students in small groups and during science practical experiments. I enjoy this work immensely and have received positive feedback regarding my teaching from the Head of Science, the pupils and their parents.

LEADERSHIP EXPERIENCE

I recognise the need for a medical student, and indeed doctor, to possess good teamworking, leadership and management skills to function effectively in such a multi-disciplinary field. My experience in this area includes:

- Activity Leader, Camp Castaway. Jun 08–Aug 08
- Captain of St Secondary School rugby team. Sept 06–Jun 07
- Head Prefect, St Secondary School. Sept 06–Jun 07

INTERESTS

I play rugby for my sixth form college in the position of flanker and have competed in several regional college tournaments. I enjoy badminton, squash and table tennis. I play the acoustic and electric guitar and have played at college functions and concerts. I enjoy cinema, reading and chess.

CAREER INTENTIONS

I have been interested in pursuing a career in medicine since beginning secondary school, after a careers awareness day. As a keen science student I have always wanted to combine my interest in biology and chemistry with a career that allows me to interact with people and I feel that medicine is such a science and art. I understand that medicine is a competitive and demanding career and have striven to increase my knowledge of and insight into my chosen field by talking to medical students and doctors, performing work experience at local hospitals and securing a job in a healthcare-related field. I am particularly drawn to Paediatrics, but am keen to experience all community and hospital specialties. I am predicted the requisite A level results for Medical School entry and feel certain I can achieve these. I believe that I have the qualities required for a good medical student; I am hard working, organised, diligent and focused and feel that I would perform well at Medical School.

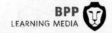

REFEREES

Mr A Teacher	**Miss B Teacher**
Headmaster	Head of Science
St Sixth Form College	St Sixth Form College
School Street	School Street
London	London
SW2 2AA	SW2 2AA
Tel: 0207 111 2222	Tel: 0207 111 2222
Email: ateacher@gmail.com	Email: bteacher@gmail.com

Chapter 3

Application for Foundation Training

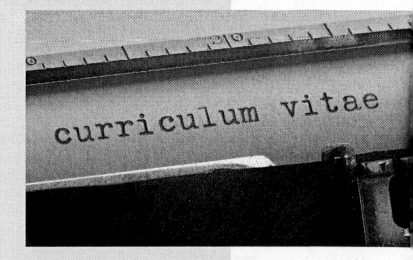

Application for Foundation Training

Introduction

You will now be reaching the final stages of your last year at Medical School. So far the biggest stressors you have faced related to your medical career involve attending lectures and placements and passing exams (no mean feat, but the really hard part is to come). As mentioned in the section pertaining to Medical School applicants, you are in a pool of tremendously high achievers, where everyone around you is at a level of competition unlike any other; and now you have actually got through Medical School, it starts to be quite tough.

By now you should be on track for passing your finals, have completed an elective and be thinking about job applications. Things have changed in medical recruitment dramatically over the last six years, and situations vary between countries and individual deaneries. Consultants often no longer get to interview their own trainees personally, much to the chagrin of many trainees and consultants. The system used to accept that if, for example, you wanted a job in Paediatrics, you could complete an optional placement with a particular consultant in that department and gain recognition as a hardworking reliable student, which would stand you in good stead come application time. Now with the introduction of various application processes such as 'matching schemes' you are usually asked to rank a list of jobs and depending on how well you fill in an application form or complete your CV, and how well you perform at a generic interview if applicable, you are ranked along with every other candidate, with the highest-scoring being offered their first choice and so on down the line. Many deaneries have ceased even to interview Foundation candidates, which has caused much controversy in the medical profession, and newer schemes by which candidates are appointed are being introduced. On the flip side however, champions of the new systems state that this has put an end to the 'old boys' nepotism

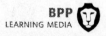

of medical students getting 'introduced' to a consultant by the relevant colleague and then 'recognised' at interview. You can debate the pros and cons endlessly, but the fact is that there are so many students now applying for Foundation jobs across the UK, that the development of a more generic system was largely inevitable. Your job is to stand out from the crowd – which is not easy when the majority of medical students follow a broad-based curriculum to prepare them for a generic Foundation job. What we say is this; the Foundation job you get is only a start to your medical career, and if you do not secure the particular Foundation rotation you ranked first, then it is not the end of the world. It is a Foundation job, to give you a platform of skills in medicine and surgery from which to launch yourself as a safe and effective doctor into the specialty you wish to pursue. Yes, it would be nice if you could get some experience in the job you want, but don't forget that a lot of you at this point will not be firmly fixed in a particular specialty and experience of other disciplines may change your mind. You may feel more strongly about what you do not want to do at this stage than what you want to do.

So if you end up with a Foundation 1 job that includes Geriatrics, Ophthalmology and Urology when you are desperate to be a GP with an interest in Psychiatry, don't worry. Use the placements you have to your advantage. Use your time wisely; think about what skills you can get during each period of the job to make you more competitive for the next. Using the example Foundation 1 rotation above, if you want to be a GP with an interest in Psychiatry, then get involved in an audit at an early stage during your geriatric job, looking at referrals to psycho-geriatrics in the community and in secondary care. Or look at the level of impotence post-transurethral resection of prostate operations and the counselling or psychiatric sexual health support available via GPs and Community Health Centres. Find a GP in the community with a similar interest and do some groundwork on what sort of things they do. All this is useful to demonstrate commitment to your specialty when asked.

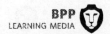

At this point, some readers will be thinking, 'I haven't a clue what I want to do yet, and how am I supposed to organise evidence of what I want to do if I don't know? Oh dear, when did it stop being fun?' Unfortunately, you are now being asked to specialise earlier and earlier, and it is somewhat unfair. A similar analogy would be to select an incredibly expensive suit after only visiting three or four shops, knowing there are more out there that you haven't perused properly. Regrettably, there is no real solution to this, and my advice is to try to see as much as possible before you are asked to decide. Speak to the Foundation 1 and 2 doctors, the specialty trainees, and look at the lifestyle of the registrars and consultants. Is this the sort of thing you can see yourself doing until you are sixty or sixty-five? If you truly don't have a clue what you want to do, then start with the rejection of what you know yourself that you dislike. For example, if you definitely know that you do not want to do surgery, then concentrate on the medical specialities, not forgetting the more 'obscure' ones like Radiology, Pathology and Public Health. There are plenty of careers fairs run by the BMJ and Royal Colleges to help you decide.

The point here is that the particular rotation you get for Foundation training is less important than the experience you gain from it. I knew a friend in my year at Medical School who ended up in the third round of jobs, not getting his first or second lot of rankings, mainly due to nerves at interview; a factor that does not always apply anymore. He ended up with a Foundation 1 job in a large district general hospital a fair distance from our university city, with a long commute, and at the time this seemed a negative thing. However, the experience and skills he took from that job made him very competitive for the round of specialty training, as the district general taught him many procedural skills such as central lines, chest drains and minor operations. Whilst in no way do I mean to suggest that medical training is a race, he is most definitely the person out of my entire group of friends that has progressed the furthest and the fastest.

In short, the applications at this point are looking for good

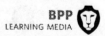

all-rounders, who may have something special on their CV, and particularly those who have shown interest in a specialty included on their chosen rotation and have made attempts to gain experience in it.

Preparation

Preparing in time for your first medical job application is very wise, and giving yourself enough time to remedy any gaps on your CV is prudent. Many students feel that the stress of Medical School is enough to cope with during their time there, but unfortunately there are now so many trainees graduating that you can no longer be 'guaranteed' a job on qualification. Medical Students have been overheard to say, 'I'm not that competitive really, so I think GP is the way forward for me'. I'm afraid that there are no 'non-competitive' specialities anymore, and GP posts were highly competitive this year. So even if that were ever true, it certainly is no longer. Hence, preparation for your final exams must also be twinned with preparation for your first job applications. Obtaining guidance regarding your CV is more difficult at this stage compared to later in your training – there is no consultant 'responsible' for you as there will be further on in your career, though some Medical Schools have a 'buddy' system in place, which provides you with a consultant contact through your medical training, though this facility is often underused and the consultant is rarely contacted. You may have become close to a particular consultant during a placement, and they may be willing to meet with you and go over your CV to identify areas that they would look for if shortlisting for a Foundation trainee. Friends that have already graduated are good sources of support, and are often only too happy to meet up and discuss applications and CVs, as they were in that position not too long ago. Try not to copy your friends' applications. This will result in dozens of very similar-looking applications and CVs being submitted or reviewed at interview, and often the experiences one person has described are not as relevant to another.

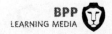

Clinical experience

Many Medical Students enjoy an elective abroad, and far from enjoying an extended holiday, most students these days apply a significant amount, if not all, of their elective period to actually doing medicine! If you have had the foresight to plan this elective in an area relating to the specialty you are applying for, well done, as this will be looked upon very favourably and elaboration regarding the specific tasks and procedures you performed there is advisable. If you did not, then think if the elective can be related to another of the specialties on the rotation you are applying for. For example, if the Foundation job you want is composed of General Surgery, Acute Medicine and Paediatrics, and it is the Acute Medicine you are particularly interested in but you spent your elective in Australia attending lots of Paediatric clinics, then you should make the most of your paediatric experience in the application.

The rest of your clinical experience will depend on the choice of your special study modules during university and the placements to which you have been assigned by the Medical School. Again, if you have decided early on which specialty you are interested in and chosen your optional modules accordingly, then the experience you will have gained here is valuable. If not then do not despair; use the final placements you have left to target the specialty you wish to pursue, attending these clinics or theatre sessions in the time available to you.

Clinical audit

It is important to understand the difference between audit and research. Audit centres on assessing a Trust's approach to a particular procedure against agreed guidance. Research aims to discover new and improved procedures. Definitions of these terms are often questions asked at interview, and application forms will try to assess your understanding of them, so be clear in your own mind what the difference between the two is. Remember the following statement:

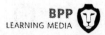

'Research involves discovering the right thing to do. Audit involves ensuring that it is done right.'

During your placements, try to involve yourself in a departmental clinical audit. It is easier to become involved in audit than research as a student, as you do not need to plan time for ethical approval and organising structured supervision; and every NHS department should be involved in clinical audit, therefore there are usually lots of them planned or currently under way at the same time.

Time pressure is obviously still a factor here, as placements are usually 6–8 weeks long, which is a relatively short space of time to get any audit project set up and completed. However, if you start this early in your placement, it is possible that you can perform the design and data collection during this period and perform the analysis and write-up later. Approach the Consultant responsible for your placement at the beginning and explain your wish to involve yourself in an audit. They may guide you towards one of the department's trainees, who might appreciate the assistance of a student in pulling together notes and filling in pro formas, and be able to help you with the rest of the audit. Keep in contact with the people you are doing work with after you move placements as it is possible that the more senior trainees will be willing to let a medical student present an audit at a meeting or help you submit it to a journal.

Clinical research

If you have performed an intercalated degree then your thesis is likely to have generated research to publish and present. It is important to keep on top of the write-up section of this work, so that when the applications roll around, you have these important papers and presentations on your CV already.

If you have not intercalated, it is certainly not expected for a trainee to be involved in research at this early stage of your career, but it is possible that during optional study modules a research

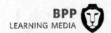

project you perform may have the mileage to be presented or published. Approach your project supervisor regarding help in this matter and they will be able to advise you.

Higher degree

If you are reading this book at an early stage in your medical student career, firstly commendations on your forward planning, and secondly, consider performing an intercalated degree such as a BSc after your third or fourth years at Medical School. In some Medical Schools this is mandatory, in others optional.

There are negatives and positives associated with an intercalated degree. A common negative cry is that an extra year at university incurs extra financial hardship (very true and difficult to reason around) and delays graduation (technically true, but only by one year, which when put in the context of a post-graduate career which could potentially last forty-three years is hardly significant). However, the medical saying 'publish or perish' has never been so significant due to the increased competition for training posts. In short, you are going to have to perform research at some stage in your career to generate the high-quality publications and presentations required for progression. It is worth considering getting involved in an interesting intercalated degree at this early stage, as the only time you will have to perform research later on is either when you are working full/part-time, or have taken time out of your career to perform a research degree. This is an opportunity to be academically very well supported in a research degree of your choosing. However, this research should be interesting to you and relevant, otherwise you will become bored, lose motivation and end up with a lower-class degree and a wasted year.

Employment

This may seem an odd section to include under 'Preparation', but with the increased financial pressure of tuition fees and student loans many students find themselves having to seek a

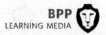

part-time or summer job to supplement their income. If this is healthcare-related then it will also be a selling point on your CV. If you are reading this in time for significant preparation, then I would suggest looking at applying for jobs related to healthcare, such as healthcare assistant or phlebotomist at your local hospital, particularly if it is a summer job that you are looking for, as combining hours with your study in the week is difficult. There are often short training courses associated with such work, but once trained and in contact with the hospital you can usually get onto a list of people willing to do weekend work, which being out-of-hours is better paid than bar-tending and will also give you some experience and skills in the work environment and some valuable material for your CV. Either contact your local hospital to enquire or look on the NHS jobs website at www.jobs.nhs.uk.

Courses

There are very few if any mandatory courses for medical students, but resuscitation courses such as Acute Life-Threatening Emergencies: Recognition and Treatment (ALERT) and Intermediate Life Support (ILS) are sometimes encouraged during the final stages of your training, to help prepare you with resuscitation skills before your Foundation 1 job. Some universities arrange the courses for their undergraduates; therefore it may be wise to find out early from your medical education centre if and when these courses are planned for you. If not, then contact the Resuscitation Training Officer at the teaching hospitals associated with your Medical School to see if these courses are available there. Alternatively, you can contact the course centres directly via their websites (ie the 'Courses' section of www.resus.org.uk). Some placements, particularly General Practice or Palliative Care, will let you attend courses that their trainees are attending, for example the Macmillan nurses run a one-day course on Breaking Bad News. Find out early in your placements if any similar courses are planned for the staff (senior nurses are often the best people to ask), and if so try to gain entry to them.

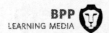

Scientific meetings/conferences

If you have performed research either through an intercalated degree or during your time in medical placements then try to make sure you submit it for presentation at a scientific meeting well in advance of the application date. This will not only give you a presentation on your CV, but attendance at an academic meeting also. Each Royal College for the relevant specialty holds career open days to give students an idea of what a career in their specialty is like, with many interesting and often famous speakers. These are possibly even more pertinent if you are not sure which career path to choose, so take advantage of them early to give yourself the best chance of making an informed choice. There are many open days at specialty Royal Colleges that are advertised through their websites and often through your own medical education centre. Attendance at these days looks favourable and shows insight and interest. There are also various committees which hold meetings such as the BMA aimed at students, which have educational and career foci and attending these will provide you with information about what is currently happening within your profession and indicate ways in which you can help or even join. This is all evidence that you are not just sitting around and waiting to graduate, but are willing to get involved with your specialty and career.

Teaching

Some of you will already have teaching experience from before you attended Medical School. Most of you will not. Again, if you are reading this early in your medical career then there are several actions you can put into motion to gain some teaching experience and skills before the applications. This is where you have an advantage compared to later on in your career. Although it may not seem it now, you have more time on your hands, as trying to gain teaching experience when working full-time is quite a stretch! At some point after the end of your pre-clinical or second years at Medical School, approach the Anatomy department and see if they need a hand with some voluntary anatomy-demonstrating during the free sessions you have in

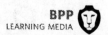

the week. As there are very few paid medical demonstrator jobs these days, it is likely that your offer of help will be very well received! This is also excellent practice for those of you who intend to become surgeons or pathologists, as the best way to consolidate your knowledge about a subject is to teach it. There is usually an Academic Consultant in charge of the medical education of junior medical students; approach them and ask if you can help to facilitate at Integrated Learning Activities or Problem Based Learning sessions. Lastly, during the summer months when most of the first- and second-year students have gone home, the unfortunate few from each year who have failed their end-of-year exams must remain for extra tuition and revision sessions before the re-sits at the end of summer. Volunteer yourself as a study-buddy via the Medical School to see if any of the junior medical students want extra help. This will not only give you some excellent material for your CV, it will introduce you to the possibility of becoming involved in medical education further down the road of your career, which is an area you may wish to involve yourself in. Make sure that you get some feedback for your teaching; this need not be any weighty graphically designed form, just a simple feedback form asking the student to outline the positive aspects of your teaching session and areas for improvement. A simple way to do this is to give each student different coloured Post-it notes and ask them to put the positive points on one colour and the suggestions for improvement on another.

Leadership/management involvement

Effective leadership and management are again two of the qualities expected of a doctor, outlined in the document *Good Medical Practice* on the GMC website. You may already have evidence of this, from your previous experience before Medical School, however recent leadership activities are what the shortlisters will be looking for. Leading in activities such as sports, student societies or being a student representative are all very good examples and can be within or outside of medicine, so if you have time before the applications, it is worth getting yourself involved in these

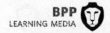

sorts of endeavours. Think outside of the box a little – have you helped to organise any charity events or social activities such as the Graduation Ball or Raising and Giving (RAG) week? Did you sit on the medical student selection panel? If not, are these areas in which you could become involved?

Logbook

During Medical School, the clinical experience that you get during your placements can vary wildly. Some people are relegated to the back of operating theatres or clinics as mere bystanders, and this is a shame. However, if you show enough enthusiasm, explain that you are keen on the specialty and ask if you can assist in procedures, then most of your supervisors will encourage you in this. They may allow you to assist and even perform some minor procedures such as suturing in A&E or theatre, removing small lesions in Dermatology or Surgery, assisting in the insertion of drains or lines in Medicine or Anaesthetics. The list goes on. If you make the effort to get involved in these things at an early stage, make a logbook. The procedure for this is explained more fully in Chapter 4 (Application for Specialty Training), but in short, ensure you record the date of the procedure, the patient's hospital number and age (but *never* their name, as removing a patient's details from the hospital environment is a serious breach of confidentiality) and the procedure you performed or assisted with. This will ensure you have a useful record with evidence to back yourself up if you are asked at interview if you have attended theatre, have inserted drains or are competent at suturing.

 Key preparation points

- Try to start preparation before the end of your final year
- Use your placements, particularly special study modules, to get involved in clinical audit or research projects. If you do, keep in touch with the team to see if it is published or presented
- Consider an intercalated degree early on in your medical career
- Find out if your Medical School will support you to attend a resuscitation course

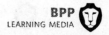

- Attend Medical Student career days and Royal college career days
- Consider taking extra time in your placements to attend clinics or events in the specialty you are interested in
- Involve yourself in formal teaching early and get feedback
- Record the procedures/operations you have performed and keep a logbook

 ## Key CV construction points

- Present information in reverse chronological order (most recent first)
- Avoid fancy fonts: ease of reading is the aim! Arial, Calibri and Cambria are personal favourites, but any font that is clear and easy to read is unlikely to offend
- Font size: no smaller than ten, twelve if possible. A shortlister that is reading dozens of CVs is likely to be irritated if having to squint
- Paragraphs: to save space, do not start a new paragraph unnecessarily
- Spacing: you will extend the length of your CV if you double-space everything. A ten-page CV is unnecessary when a four-page version would suffice
- 'I': avoid the use of the word 'I', as it can become very repetitive
- Length: historically the 'keep to two pages' rule has been applied. Less than five and more than one is recommended
- Alignment: try to keep everything symmetrical, consistent and in alignment. There are fancy computer programs that can do this for you, but a keen eye, printing out a test copy and looking at it carefully will achieve the same result
- Bold and underlining: avoid overuse. Use headings to highlight areas of importance and use the bold function sparingly, eg for your surname on any publications. Do not be tempted to mix and match bold and underlining throughout your CV, as it will cause confusion. Stick to one
- Bullet points can be very useful to summarise information clearly and succinctly, but do not overuse them
- Acronyms: as an individual responsible for shortlisting may be from a different specialty, avoid the use of acronyms

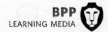

Writing the CV

Personal/professional details

Include your full name, address (make this a reliable address if you are likely to be moving home before the interviews, or make sure you have mail redirection in plenty of time) and telephone numbers (at least work and mobile); BMA number if appropriate and Medical Indemnity Membership number. For ease of reading and conservation of space, keep your contact and personal details on the left and your professional details on the right (see example at the end of the chapter). Ensure you include a professional-sounding email account, as a non-professional one such as Wildman69@hotmail.com, does not project the right image.

Qualifications and prizes/distinctions

Always include the university/professional body from which your qualifications were gained and the dates. State the start and completion dates of your medical degree and any prizes or distinctions you have achieved so far. If you completed an intercalated degree, or have read a degree prior to starting Medical School, provide a short summary of the course/subject. It is still acceptable to state your GCSE and A level results at this stage of training, but do not list them exhaustively (see example).

Employment

If you have performed a part-time or full-time job either prior to starting your Medical Training or during your time at Medical School, and the qualities that position required relate to those desired in medicine, then state your experience briefly here. It obviously helps if this work is healthcare-related (eg cardiac technician, staff nurse, support worker for the hospital/elderly/ disabled) and requires good communication, sensitivity and respect for patients. But experience in other areas of work can emphasise what skills and attributes you have already acquired in the workplace. Holding down a part-time job at Medical

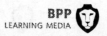

School can be demanding, but shows you are hard-working and can organise your time well. Experience with a part-time job working at the university bar or in a call centre (to give two real-life examples from our own experience) can attest to your organisational, time-management and diplomacy skills, and candidates are asked about this. The most important thing is to emphasise that the employment experience you have is relevant to what you are applying for – the current buzzword for this is 'transferable skills.'

Courses

If you have completed any courses related to medicine during Medical School, for example resuscitation, mental health, dealing with disfigurement, etc, then list them here with their dates (in reverse chronological order) and also the location and course provider (eg the Resuscitation Council for ILS.).

Clinical experience

Summarising the clinical experience you have gained during Medical School is recommended and can help the individual shortlisting to see that you have been earnest in the acquisition of knowledge and skills needed to become a competent doctor. Having said that, do not exaggerate! Stating that you are fully competent to remove an appendix is likely to arouse deep suspicion, even if your consultant did take you through the procedure several times. Refer to the person specification and briefly match your experience to what is expected at this stage, but include anything above and beyond that you have managed to achieve. For example:

> *My clinical years at Medical School have given me a broad-based experience in medicine, surgery and General Practice. I have received excellent feedback from consultants supervising my placements and have passed all my assessments to a high level. I am competent in taking histories and performing clinical examinations, initiating investigations and management. I have*

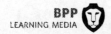

experience in venepuncture, intravenous cannulation, ECG interpretation and taking arterial blood gases. I have taken time to shadow Foundation trainees in all aspects of their jobs to increase the knowledge and skills that will be required of me at the end of my medical student training. As I am particularly interested in Paediatrics, I have performed my optional study module with the Paediatric cardiology consultants, attended ward rounds and clinics and involved myself in the departmental audit to further improve my knowledge of this specialty.

Clinical audit

If you have managed to become involved in an audit as a medical student at any level, then include a brief summary of the audit and your role in the process. If you were supported in leading the audit, then certainly state that, but do not be tempted to exaggerate your involvement. Try to emphasise your knowledge of the importance and process of clinical audit, describing the stages you were personally involved in, the result of the audit and its implications for the audit team in terms of practice. Remember that clinical audit is a cyclical process and the need to close the audit loop. For example:

> *As part of my attachment to the respiratory team, I was involved in a departmental audit into the antibiotic prescriptions for patients with Chronic Obstructive Airways Disease. With the ST2 doctor for my firm, I performed a literature review, identified local hospital prescribing guidance and helped collect data from case notes and discharge summaries. The results of the audit showed that local guidance was not being followed in over 25% of cases, and action was taken to insert local antibiotic prescribing guidance in the departmental handbook. I attended the regional audit day where this audit was presented by my ST2 co-author, and a further audit is planned in a year to ensure compliance with guidance has improved and to close the audit loop.*

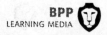

Research experience

If you have been involved in a research project at any stage, either as part of an intercalated degree or during a placement at Medical School, then provide a brief description of the project and your role in the research team. If you have significant experience of research prior to attending Medical School then it is acceptable to provide a similar summary, but in reverse chronological order, with Medical School projects first. Provide details of the dissemination of results, whether publication or presentation. For example:

> *As part of my optional attachment in Obstetrics and Gynaecology, I was involved in a research project looking at the outcomes following vaginal prolapse repair surgery with colposuspension. Along with the Consultant and Registrar supervising my attachment, I performed a comprehensive literature search, and helped design a data collection pro forma. I collected and analysed case notes, and attended follow-up clinics for patients where I helped to assess symptoms of urinary incontinence using a validated questionnaire, the results of which were compared with pre-operative scores identified retrospectively. The results showed that patients who had undergone this procedure had a statistically significant improvement in symptoms. My co-author presented our findings at the Regional Teaching Day and the paper has been submitted for publication in the British Journal of Obstetrics and Gynaecology.*

Publications

If you have any publications, prior to or during Medical School, then list them here in reverse chronological order. As explained in later chapters, there are many ways to reference publications, and it is acceptable to use any style you are familiar with. I prefer the Harvard style, which is used in the CV example below. Ensure your name appears in the right place in the list of contributors, correctly reflecting the extent of your contribution, and highlight it in bold to allow it to be seen easily. If you have more than one publication (well done!) then see Chapter 4 for details of

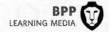

how to divide your publications into different categories, ie full manuscripts, case reports, etc.

Presentations

If you have presented a case report, audit or research then list your presentations here. Split them into categories of hierarchy, the most prestigious first for example, International Presentations, then National, then Regional. Within those categories, still follow the reverse chronological order rule (see the example below for guidance). Presentations do not have to be referenced like publications, but all relevant details still need to be included such as the date, venue and title, again ensuring your name is in the appropriate order and highlighted in bold. As explained in more detail in Chapter 4, it is acceptable to list presentations where you have been involved in the work, as long as you ensure the presenter's name is first when listing the authors.

Scientific meetings/conferences

List any conferences or meetings you have attended in reverse chronological order with the title, dates and place of the meeting.

Teaching

If you have any formal teaching experience prior to starting Medical School, for example if you are a mature student and have experience of teaching inside or outside of the medical field, then describe your role here. Equally, if whilst at Medical School you became involved in teaching, formal or otherwise, describe it briefly and include the dates the teaching was delivered over. Remember, it is important to have some evidence of your teaching, such as student feedback or formal letters, to present at interview if required. Include a short statement, which will let the shortlisters know that you are aware of the requirements of a doctor to have skills in teaching. For example:

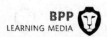

During Medical School I became very interested in teaching junior students and enjoy this aspect of medicine immensely. My experience in teaching includes:

- *Formal Anatomy teaching to medical students – Glasgow University, Dec 2007 to present*
- *Volunteer assistant Spanish teacher to Community College Evening students – Glasgow, Aug 2008 to present*
- *Teaching English to school students during my gap year- Peru, Aug 04–Feb 05*

Leadership/management involvement

List all roles of leadership, positions of responsibility or management that you have been involved in. Include the dates to which this applies and a brief summary of the position and your role. Avoid listing school/sixth form college responsibilities here. (Saying that you were a head prefect, whilst fine for your medical student applications, looks a bit lacklustre five years down the line.) Similarly to above, highlight your awareness of the management and leadership skills needed for a medical career. This does not need to be at the start of your experience, and can be slotted into your explanation of your role. For example:

Medical Student Representative for International Week, Glasgow, April 2005

This position involved six months' organisation and co-ordination of events for the celebration of international culture and cuisine. I led a team of people in this event and it was well received by all who attended, including the Dean of the Medical School. This experience improved my teamworking, leadership and management skills, which I feel are essential for a doctor. We raised over two thousand pounds for the International charity UNICEF.

Personal interests

The inclusion of a 'Personal interests' section allows the individuals shortlisting to see that you do have a life outside

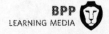

of Medical School, involving yourself with activities other than revising and going to your placements. This has gained increased emphasis over the years, as it is generally thought that doctors with hobbies and interests are less likely to suffer from stress at work. If these interests support or develop skills that are desirable in the workplace then this is obviously of relevance to your career and if you have achieved goals in these interests then this gives evidence to your commitment. For example, involvement in team activities such as sports or societies, creative interests such as art and theatre, or studies in foreign languages or music are all relevant. As I will mention in later chapters, be honest when listing your interests because it is easy to be caught in a lie and this would raise questions about your trustworthiness as a person and as a doctor. Also, be selective in the interests that you list, bearing in mind the still very conservative nature of medicine. A list of musical festivals you have attended to expand your experience of popular music is unlikely to impress.

Additional experience and career intentions

If there are any areas of experience that you have not already mentioned in your CV that you think are relevant to your skills and experience and show you as a good candidate, then list them briefly here. This could include experience you have gained on your elective and gap year, or any optional attachments you have completed that have not already been mentioned. If you have performed any additional work such as shadowing seniors out-of-hours or volunteer/charity work, then include a summary of it here. Anything that may make you stand out or demonstrate that you have made the effort to gain additional experience will be looked upon favourably. A short statement of your career intentions is also advised, to give your CV direction, but staying relatively non-specific is also advised here, as it is a generic Foundation job you are applying for. Whilst you may be absolutely certain you want to be a Forensic Pathologist, it may be wise to indicate your interest gently whilst referring to gaining experience in other fields as part of your Foundation

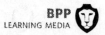

year, so as not to seem too rigid in your career choices before you have even started your working life.

Referees

The referees you select at this point must come from the consultants you have met whilst on Medical Student placement. There are usually one or two consultants who have stood out as being particularly supportive to you during your clinical years at Medical School, who would support your applications. If you have a particular post or specialty in mind at this stage, then try to select a consultant from that specialty. Make sure that you ask them well in advance if they would be happy to act as a referee, as it is considered very rude just to put their names down and expect them to fill in a reference with no prior notice. It may also be wise to meet them personally for this, contacting their secretary to explain your position and arrange a time when you could come to see them. This will benefit you in two ways. Firstly, it will show them that you have made the effort to come and speak to them personally about being a referee, which is more courteous than sending an email or leaving a telephone message. Secondly, it will remind them who you are – most consultants see hundreds of medical students each year, but they are likely to remember the ones who took time to come and request a reference personally. Bring a copy of your CV to this meeting, as consultants often refer to it when writing a reference.

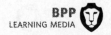

Example CV for application to Foundation Training

John James Smith

Date of birth:	1 January 1984	**BMA:**	200000
Nationality:	British	**MPS:**	300000
Address:	12 Willow Drive, Glasgow G1 1AA		
Telephone:	0151 222 5555 / 0777333000		
E-mail:	jjsmith@doctors.org.uk		

QUALIFICATIONS

2003–Present	**University of Glasgow**	MBChB
1995–2002	**St Secondary School, London**	4 A levels Grade A 10 GCSEs Grade A–B

EMPLOYMENT

Aug 02–Feb 03   Support Worker, Winnersh, Berkshire NHS Trust

In this role, along with other members of the care team, I was responsible for the home support of adults with physical and learning disabilities in their home environment and in the community. I provided personal care, accompanied them to physical therapy and hospital appointments and also in their day-to-day leisure activities.

CLINICAL EXPERIENCE

My clinical years at Medical School have given me a broad-based experience in medicine, surgery and General Practice. I have received excellent feedback from consultants supervising my placements and have passed all my assessments to a high level. I am competent in taking histories and performing clinical examinations, initiating investigations and management. I have experience in venepuncture, intravenous cannulation, ECG interpretation and taking arterial

---

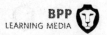

blood gases. I have taken time to shadow Foundation trainees in all aspects of their job to increase the knowledge and skills that will be required of me at the end of my Medical Student training. As I am particularly interested in Obstetrics and Gynaecology, I performed my optional study modules with the Obstetric and Gynaecology teams at Glasgow Royal Infirmary, attending ward rounds and clinics and involving myself in the departmental audit to improve my knowledge of this specialty further.

COURSES

A.L.E.R.T. Course	Resus. Council, Paisley	Dec 07
ILS Course	Resus. Council, Glasgow	Sept 07

RESEARCH EXPERIENCE

Outcomes following vaginal prolapse repair. Consultant, A. Registrar, B. **Smith, J.**

As part of my optional attachment in Obstetrics and Gynaecology, I was involved in a research project looking at the outcomes following vaginal prolapse repair surgery with colposuspension. Along with the Consultant and Registrar supervising my attachment, I performed a comprehensive literature search, and helped design a data collection pro forma. I collected and analysed case notes and attended follow-up clinics for patients where I helped to assess symptoms of urinary incontinence using a validated questionnaire, the results of which were compared with pre-operative scores identified retrospectively. The results showed that patients who had undergone this procedure had a statistically significant improvement in symptoms. This paper has been submitted for publication in the British Journal of Obstetrics and Gynaecology.

PRESENTATIONS

Regional

Audit of antibiotic prescribing in patients with chronic obstructive airways disease. Doctor, A. **Smith, J.** Consultant, A. Respiratory Services Regional Audit Day, Glasgow Royal Infirmary, Glasgow, Dec 2007.

SCIENTIFIC MEETINGS/CONFERENCES ATTENDED

The National Trainee Surgeons Meeting	London Jul 05

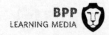

CLINICAL AUDIT

Audit of antibiotic prescribing in patients with Chronic Obstructive Airways Disease. Doctor, A. **Smith, J.** Consultant, A. Glasgow Royal Infirmary, Glasgow, Dec 2007.

As part of my attachment to the respiratory team, I was involved in a departmental audit into the antibiotic prescriptions for patients with Chronic Obstructive Airways Disease. With the ST2 doctor for my firm, I performed a literature review, identified local hospital prescribing guidance and helped collect data from case notes and discharge summaries. The results of the audit showed that local guidance was not being followed in over 25% of cases, and action was taken to insert local antibiotic prescribing guidance into the departmental handbook. I attended the regional audit day where this audit was presented by my ST2 co-author, and a further audit is planned in a year to ensure compliance with guidance has improved and to close the audit loop.

TEACHING

During Medical School I became very interested in teaching junior students and enjoy this aspect of medicine immensely. My experience in teaching includes:

*   Volunteer assistant Spanish teacher to Community College Evening students – Glasgow, Aug 2008 to present.

*   Formal Anatomy teaching to medical students – Glasgow University, Dec 2007 to present.

*   Teaching English to school students during my Gap year – Peru, Aug 04–Feb 05.

LEADERSHIP AND MANAGEMENT EXPERIENCE

Medical Student Representative for International Week, Glasgow, April 2005

This position involved six months' organisation and co-ordination of events for the celebration of international culture and cuisine. I led a team of people in this event and it was well received by all who attended including the Dean of the Medical School. This experience improved my teamworking, leadership and management skills, which I feel are essential for a doctor in the workplace. We raised over two thousand pounds for the International charity UNICEF.

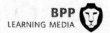

PERSONAL INTERESTS

I enjoy tennis and swimming, and have passed my Grade 6 piano examination. I am fluent in Spanish and volunteer at my local community college helping to teach beginners' evening classes.

ADDITIONAL EXPERIENCE AND CAREER INTENTIONS

During my elective in Madrid, Spain, I was attached to a large teaching hospital. I involved myself in all activities with the Spanish junior doctors, including rounds, clinics, theatre and teaching. I organised an attachment to the Royal Maternity Hospital in Madrid, and gained valuable insight into the differences in pathology, treatment and outlook of the Spanish Obstetrics Services and I am very grateful for the experience that this elective afforded.

I have always enjoyed teaching, and during my Gap year in Peru, I taught English at several schools in the hill tribe areas, This experience strengthened my desire to be involved in teaching in the medical field, something that I have continued during Medical School as a volunteer teacher for junior medical students in Anatomy and exam revision sessions.

I am particularly interested in a career in Obstetrics and Gynaecology and have striven to gain additional experience in order to gain insight and knowledge of this field. I have shadowed trainees in several areas of their practice, attended clinics out-of-hours and performed all of my optional attachments within the field of Obstetrics and Gynaecology, helping with research projects. I am looking forward to the challenges and experiences that my Foundation year will offer, and am confident that I will be a safe, competent and efficient Foundation trainee and member of the healthcare team.

REFEREES

Mr A Consultant
Consultant Obstetrician
Princess Royal Maternity Unit,
GRI
Castle Street
Glasgow
G4 0SF
Tel: 0141 111 2222 ext 1111
Email: aconsultant@ggc.nhs.uk

Miss B Consultant
Consultant Gynecologist
Princess Royal Maternity Unit,
GRI
Castle Street
Glasgow
G4 0SF
Tel: 0141 222 3333 ext 2222
Email: bconsultant@ggc.nhs.uk

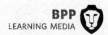

Chapter 4

Application for Specialty Training

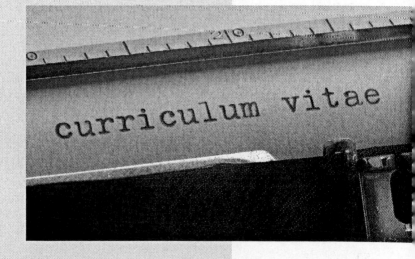

Application for Specialty Training

Introduction

If you are applying for Specialty Training, which now combines the old system of basic and higher training, then you are probably at one of three stages:

- You are still in your Foundation 2 year and are now coming to apply for a specialty at the initial stage of run-through Specialty Training (ST1 year) or a two-year initial-level Core Training (CT1/2)

- You have finished the 'Core Training' of initial Specialist training (CT1/2) and are now applying for the intermediate level Specialty Training (ST3)

- You have spent a year or so after your Foundation years (or equivalents) in a 'fixed term' Specialist training appointment (FTSTA), staff-grade post or research job and are trying to enter Specialist training at an initial/intermediate level (ST2 or ST3 years)

All of this seems incredibly confusing because at present, as explained in the Introduction, the medical profession is in a state of change. Across the UK there have been different job titles for specialty training at different levels aimed at trainees with various levels of experience. Regardless of the titles, the aim of these jobs is to provide a platform of knowledge in whichever specialty you choose, from which you can build upon to make yourself skilled and competitive to progress through your training to consultant level.

Regardless of the level you are looking to enter Specialist training at, the experience you have gained over the last seven-plus years will help you on your quest for your chosen career. Entry to Specialty Training is incredibly competitive at any level and with reductions in national training numbers and de-coupling of the initial and intermediate stages of Specialty Training likely to continue, it is probable that this will increase. Therefore you must use the time you have in whatever post you are currently in, to maximise your chances of being selected for interview. All specialties are looking for evidence on your CV and application form that you have carefully considered this choice of specialty, understand what it involves and if possible have gained some experience in it.

If you are applying for initial Specialty Training (ST1/CT1), by now you should have achieved your basic Foundation competencies, completed courses relevant to your training and performed at least one clinical audit. The transition from generic Foundation doctor to Specialty trainee is daunting, as it suddenly seems as if the stakes have been raised. The key difference between the application for your first medical Foundation job and that for Specialty Training, is that you will now be expected to demonstrate relevant clinical competencies (not usually a problem if you are on course to pass your Foundation years), audit experience, courses and possibly professional exams.

If you are applying for intermediate Specialty Training (ST3), you should have evidence of progression over the year/s since your Foundation or equivalent years, with more evidence of clinical competencies, more than one clinical audit, completion of courses relevant to your stage of training, and some evidence of research experience. You should preferably also have passed some parts of your chosen specialty's Royal College examinations.

As with all applications, the way to structure your CV is to present the information required clearly and logically, so that the individuals shortlisting or interviewing can quickly see the evidence of skills and experience that pertain to your application. The difference at this stage is that you must tailor it to reflect the skills, experience and attributes required for a medical doctor, GP or surgeon as stipulated in the job description, level-specific person specification and selection criteria of the role. This is not difficult to do, as all Foundation training must include elements of surgery and

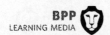

medicine, and more experienced trainees that are applying for intermediate Specialty Training will have a Foundation equivalent and further experience on top of this. However, preparation can go a long way. If you are applying to a more 'specialist' specialty, for example Paediatrics, Radiology, Psychiatry or Public Health, then knowledge and evidence relating to your experience within the chosen specialty is even more important.

Preparation

As discussed previously, with the best will in the world a CV guide cannot give you the actual material and content to put on your CV; this is down to the hard work and commitment you have shown since Medical School. Early planning of how to improve and develop your CV for a given post is well advised and a friendly consultant is invaluable in this quest. Approach your consultant, particularly your educational supervisor, with a copy of your CV and ask if they will go through it with you to see where there are areas you could improve. Most consultants will be happy to do this, as they will remember their own anguish when trying to secure a particular position.

If there are gaps in your CV after your previous positions, then take steps to remedy this as quickly as possible. These steps can be relatively easy (eg expand outside interests, book on to relevant courses, involve yourself in an audit) or may require more commitment (volunteer to teach anatomy/physiology at the University, book a college exam and start revising, register for a distance learning qualification). Some of these steps take more time than others to complete, and it depends on how committed you are to following that specialty, and how much time you have before the application deadline, as to what you can achieve. However, do not despair! Print out a copy of your CV. Look at it critically and honestly. Compare yourself with your peers and their achievements, as unfortunately these are the people you are competing with. If there are large gaps in your CV, think practically with the resources you have and the time left that you have to prepare.

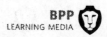

Clinical experience

If you have been lucky enough to have a post in your chosen specialty as part of your Foundation programme or have completed an FTSTA or staff grade post in your specialty, then this will help towards the acquisition of specialty-specific skills and experience. Unfortunately, if this is not the case you will have to put a bit more work in. If you already have contacts within the field of your choice, then get in touch with them as early as possible to arrange a period of shadowing. If you do not already know someone in the specialty, contact a consultant, usually the Clinical Director of the department, via his secretary and arrange a meeting to express your desire to gain experience in this field before the specialty applications commence. Most consultants will be impressed at the foresight and level of commitment this requires and will be more than happy to help. Some departments are happy to let you take up to five days of study leave in your current post to perform a clinical attachment in a different specialty, but I am afraid this is very dependent on the goodwill of the department you are working for. If not, a few days of annual leave may need to be sacrificed to perform this shadowing. Try to attend a range of clinics, ward rounds and theatres or procedures, so that you may display a comprehensive level of shadowing.

Clinical audit

This is definitely feasible, as all Foundation trainees need to perform at least one audit as part of their training and many specialties have areas of overlap, which you can use to your advantage. For example, an FTSTA2 doctor undertaking four months in A&E who wishes to pursue a career in General Surgery may look to perform an audit in abdominal trauma – comparing ATLS guidance to standards. Or a Foundation doctor working in general practice, who desires to secure a medical job in Rheumatology, would find it easy to audit the patients in their practice on a disease-modifying drug such as methotrexate, comparing their practice against national guidelines for blood tests or tertiary reviews. Or a Core Medical Trainee wishing

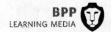

to work in Psychiatry could look at the number of patients admitted with overdose and audit the suicide risk questions performed in A&E or the community follow-up after discharge. The list is endless. By doing this early, you will find that when the application deadline for the next job opportunity comes around, you will have a relevant piece of work to present on your CV and discuss at interview. You can talk to your educational supervisor regarding the choice of audit; they usually have some good ideas and there will always be a registrar keen to supervise you. However, do not get railroaded into performing audits or research into subjects that are not relevant to your area of interest.

If you complete an audit – present it, even if this is at your hospital morbidity and mortality meeting or audit day! There is absolutely no point in performing the audit if you do not share the results with your colleagues. In fact, if you do not disseminate the results of your audit then you are not complying with General Medical Council guidance regarding this matter, as the sharing of information generated from clinical audit and research is part of Good Medical Practice. Presenting your work will not only mean you are promoting best practice, but also improving your presentation skills and securing another presentation for inclusion in your CV. If you have written your work up, then submit it for publication. This seems very daunting at first, but a good registrar is invaluable here, as they will have prior experience of this and will be able to advise you regarding the most suitable journal to submit to, help you or give advice regarding the write up and referencing and guide you on the practicalities of submission. If they have helped you significantly with the audit, remember to put their name after yours in the author list! The worst-case scenario is that the paper is rejected, and there are plenty of other journals to try if this is the case. Yes, it's time-consuming, but the value of including a publication in your CV forever will make it all worthwhile.

Clinical research

As mentioned in Chapter 3 (Application for Foundation Training) it is important to make sure you understand the difference between audit and research. Clinical audit compares current practice with best standards whereas research asks questions and aims to find answers.

Research projects usually take a fair amount of time to set up, particularly if they are prospective and will involve any form of ethical approval. Trainees applying for intermediate Specialty Training may have some experience of this already and you often need a fair amount of help and supervision. However, do not let this deter you if you have a good idea – think of what value it will provide for the next job application after this one! Remember, clinical research does not have to involve you shutting yourself away in a laboratory for endless hours. There are plenty of ward-based or patient-focussed projects that you can get involved in if you can't face being away from patient contact. However, if you cannot think of any research ideas then approach your Consultant or Registrar and see if they have any. Often there will be a research project in progress that they are keen to finish but may need some work on statistics, writing up, etc. Do not let statistics deter you either – hospitals associated with universities usually have a very knowledgeable and friendly medical statistician who would be happy to give you advice. If you do not have access to a statistician then *Essential Medical Statistics* by Kirkwood and Sterne (2003) is an excellent book outlining clinically relevant examples.

Higher degree

Again, this is something to start planning early, particularly as the completion of part-time courses can be spread over a longer time period, but starting these now may be useful for your consultant applications. Think of it in terms of when it will be finished to put on your CV. For example, if you are a Foundation 2 doctor starting a three-year part-time MSc, you will finish the course in time for it to be on your CV for applications for intermediate

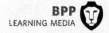

Specialty Training (ST3). It is perfectly reasonable to include in your CV that you have registered for these courses or degrees, or indeed started it; this will indicate interest and commitment to the subject. Examples could include an MSc or MA in science subjects or Medical Education.

Courses

Practically every trainee, whichever stage they are at, will have completed the mandatory courses required for their level and while it is important to have these, it is useful to think outside of the box. Are there some smaller and inexpensive courses that you could attend? Good examples are locally run courses on subjects like breaking bad news or dealing with mental health issues. Your hospital and postgraduate medical education centre should be a good place to look for these. Selection criteria based on person specifications usually award specific points for certain courses completed, eg ALS/ATLS, teaching or management. Look at the person specification for the level you are applying to. These can be found in the online section for Specialty Training on the relevant MMC websites in the UK. The Royal College website of your chosen specialty will have a list of the courses run targeted at your particular specialty, though be advised these can be expensive and must be relevant to your level. There is no point in turning up at an advanced facial aesthetics course if you have not attended a basic surgical skills course. Courses provided by private companies can also add value to your CV but it is important to ensure they are Continual Professional Development (CPD) accredited and delivered by an experienced facilitator.

Membership exams

Whichever specialty you choose, you will not be able to escape the relevant Royal College exams. Some of you will already have started these, if not completed them already. Think practically about the effort and commitment these exams require and give yourself time to revise, as it is expensive, not to mention incredibly disheartening, to re-take. If you have a job that involves a lighter

58

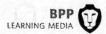

workload or rota commitment than the rest, it may be wise to plan your revision time around this to increase your chances of success. If you are very well prepared, you may be adding an exam pass to your CV before your applications!

Scientific meetings and conferences

This is probably more relevant to applicants for intermediate Specialty Training, but if you have presented any work at meetings then you have often attended the whole meeting, so include it in your CV. Attendance at scientific meetings takes planning, you often have to apply for study leave and organise transport and/or accommodation, but it is a good way to show your level of commitment and that you are interested in the current evidence available in your specialty. Find out about these meetings early, the secretary of the Clinical Director of your department is a good source of information, as emails regarding these days usually come through them. Also there are plenty of meetings aimed at more junior trainees such as various specialty societies, Royal College open days or career open days that can be added to this section to give evidence of your commitment and interest in your intended specialty. Think back and see if you can remember attending some of these in the past, even at Medical School.

Teaching

Very few jobs now involve anatomy demonstration or teaching at a formal level, so evidence of formal teaching experience is difficult to provide. However, many specialty person specifications at all levels of training award extra points to those applicants who have made the effort to involve themselves in teaching. For more senior applicants, try to find out if there are any courses being run or promoted by your department, and if appropriate (ie not a course for those more experienced than yourself!) offer to help teach or present something, as this is evidence of formal teaching experience. Attendance at a formal teaching skills course can also help to improve your application, and many deaneries run courses like 'Teaching the Teachers' or 'Doctor

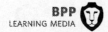

as Teacher' for Foundation level/Specialty trainees. If possible, try to arrange with your Anatomy department a few sessions of volunteer teaching to medical students. Offering to help with mock exams and clinical skills centres might be worthwhile also. If you are going to conduct informal teaching then try to ensure you gain some form of feedback for this in terms of a feedback form or suggestion notes.

Logbook

Whatever specialty you have chosen to pursue, the procedures you perform during your time in Foundation training and beyond are core skills that you may continue to use during your progression through Specialty Training. For example, chest drains for medics, lumbar punctures for paediatricians, minor operations for surgeons, fracture manipulation for orthopaedics, central/arterial lines for anaesthetists etc. Not everyone will gain all of these skills early so make sure that if you are fortunate enough to have done some, that you can provide evidence of this. Therefore, record these in a logbook *as you go along*. It is very irritating to have to spend a long time looking for the details of a patient you performed a procedure on six months ago. Some of you will already have a comprehensive logbook, but for those of you who do not, logbook formats are available in most online specialty portfolios, and for surgical trainees there are the Intercollegiate Surgical Curriculum Programme logbooks online (www.iscp.ac.uk) and the pan-surgical elogbook (www.elogbook.org). If there is not a specific logbook available for your specialty then creating a hospital-based logbook with password protection is possible by talking to your IT department – this is to ensure patient confidentiality. Numbers and ages, but *not* names and dates of birth, must identify all patients.

Key preparation points

- Prepare as early as possible
- Conduct a specialty-relevant audit during your Foundation Training/Core Training/Fixed term job. Write it up, present it and submit it for meetings/journals

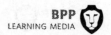

- Consider applying for a distance learning higher degree such as an MSc or Postgraduate Diploma
- Attend mandatory courses and any optional extra specialty-relevant courses
- Consider attending scientific specialty meetings and 'open days' relevant to your level of training
- Consider commencing or completing your membership exams
- Shadow a Core or Specialty trainee in the specialty you are hoping to pursue
- Keep a record of any formal teaching you have delivered together with any volunteer teaching to junior trainees and students, ensuring you get feedback
- Book on to a teaching skills course
- Record the procedures/operations you have performed and keep a logbook

 ## Key CV construction points

- Always present information in reverse chronological order (most recent first). The most recent things you have done are of most interest to the individuals shortlisting you. Do not hide them amongst your A levels or a project you did in first year at Medical School
- Avoid fancy fonts: ease of reading is the aim. Arial, Calibri and Cambria are personal favourites, but any font that is clear and easy to read is unlikely to offend
- Font size: no smaller than ten, twelve if possible. A shortlister that is reading dozens of CVs is likely to be irritated if having to squint
- Paragraphs: to save space, do not start a new paragraph unnecessarily
- Spacing: you will extend the length of your CV if you double-space everything. A ten-page CV is unnecessary when a four-page version would suffice
- 'I': avoid the use of the word 'I' as it can become very repetitive
- Length: historically the 'keep to two pages' rule has been applied. Less than five and more than one is recommended, as it will depend on the amount of experience you have to include in your CV
- Alignment: try to keep everything symmetrical, consistent and in alignment. There are fancy computer programs that can do this for you, but a keen eye, printing out a test copy and looking at it carefully will achieve the same result

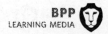

- Bold/underlining: avoid overuse. Employ headings to highlight areas of importance, and use the bold function sparingly, eg for your surname against any publications. However, do not be tempted to mix and match bold and underlining throughout your CV, as it will cause confusion. Stick to one
- Bullet points can be very useful to summarise information clearly and succinctly, but do not overuse them
- Acronyms: as an individual responsible for shortlisting may be from a different specialty, avoid the use of acronyms

Writing the CV

Personal/professional details

Include your full name, address and telephone numbers (at least work and mobile) as well as your GMC number, BMA number if appropriate and Medical Indemnity Membership number. For ease of reading and conservation of space, keep your contact and personal details on the left and your professional details on the right (see the example provided later in this chapter).

Qualifications and prizes/distinctions

Always include the University/professional body from which your qualifications were gained, and the dates. If you are currently studying towards taking a higher degree or indeed have completed one at Medical School, provide a short summary of the course/subject. Any prizes or distinctions achieved at Medical School or beyond, particularly if they pertain to your specialty interest, should be included here. Avoid putting GCSE and A level results at this stage of training, as they will take up space and are unlikely to earn any extra points, as the majority of individuals within medicine achieved high numbers of As and A*s. Also include here your completion of any parts of Royal College membership exams undertaken.

Employment

As most applications are due early in the calendar year, it is possible (and a common grumble amongst trainees), that if you

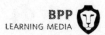

are on a rotation you will have completed only one of your Foundation 2/Core Training jobs. Include future employment, particularly if it involves posts within the specialty or relating to the specialty to which you are applying. List your current employment next and then your previous jobs with the inclusive grade, specialty and hospital in reverse chronological order, with the most recent first. If you are currently on a Core Training or Fixed Term Specialty Training Rotation, make this clear in your listing of previous employment, so that shortlisters can see that you have already secured a competitive job (see example).

Courses

List courses with their dates (in reverse chronological order as always) and also the location and course provider, eg Royal College of Surgeons for ATLS and the Resuscitation Council for ALS.

Clinical experience

A brief statement of your clinical experience can help the individual shortlisting to focus on any particularly relevant skills and experience you have achieved over the past two years. Try not to dwell too much on the achievement of basic competencies. Again, refer to the person specification and briefly summarise what is expected at this stage but include anything above and beyond that you have managed to achieve. For example a Foundation trainee might put:

My Foundation rotations have allowed me to develop and improve skills related to Anaesthetics. I have received positive competency-based feedback regarding my Foundation performance in clinical skills via structured assessment tools. I am competent in the assessment and management of the severely ill patient and have performed arterial line insertion under supervision and assisted in central line insertion, as evidenced by my logbook. I have taken time to shadow senior Anaesthetic and ICU colleagues in both elective and emergency practice to increase my knowledge and experience.

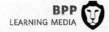

Whereas an applicant for intermediate Specialty Training (ST3) may write:

> *My training rotations in Accident and Emergency medicine have given me a broadly based experience of the specialties allied to A&E and ample opportunity to develop my clinical and procedural skills. I am competent in the assessment and management of most medical and surgical emergencies presenting to A&E and have received positive competency-based feedback as evidence for this. I am skilled in intubation and the maintenance of anaesthesia, insertion of central lines, fracture manipulation, joint relocation, burns assessment and resuscitation, and have gained considerable paediatric skill by shadowing my senior colleagues at the Children's Hospital to increase my knowledge and experience.*

Clinical audit

Audit is not only mandatory, it is very popular at the moment due to the prominence of Continuing Professional Development and Clinical Governance, so if you have been involved in audits then expand on them, particularly if there are gaps in other areas of your CV. Do not include a synopsis of the whole audit, but a brief overview of the subject, the guidance around which your audit standards were developed and your role in the audit. If you were the lead in the audit, then say so. Good words to use are 'initiated', 'led', and 'presented'. Describe the stages of the audit to inform the person creating the shortlist that you were involved at every stage and that you recognise the essential steps of audit. For example:

> *I initiated this audit, which looked at the complications suffered and the length of stay associated with appendicectomy performed in our unit. I performed a literature review, identifying national guidance, collected data using a pro forma I had designed and performed statistical analysis. Our results were compared to national standards and found to be above acceptable. The results of this audit were presented at our departmental audit meeting*

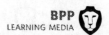

and a further audit is planned in a year's time to ensure we are maintaining standards and closing the audit loop.

Never forget the importance of presenting the findings and closing the audit loop! If your unit's results are not up to the agreed standards, then say what changes are planned and when the re-audit is to take place.

Research experience

The inclusion of a section detailing your experience in research projects should be considered, particularly if you are lacking in publications and presentations at this stage, and there are interesting projects in which you have been involved but have not yet been published or presented. This can help you highlight your understanding of the research process to the shortlisters and show that you have been involved in research at a Foundation level. Ensure that you include a statement regarding your intent to submit the project for presentation or publication, in line with good practice. As with clinical audit, the summaries should include a brief overview including the type of research, concentrating on your involvement in the project and the outcome of the research. Another good point to insert into your description is an awareness of the need for maintenance of confidentiality when performing research projects, and this is sometimes a question asked at interview. For example:

> *I designed and performed this retrospective study into revision surgery performed for ankle fracture non-union. Under senior guidance I performed a literature search, designed a pro forma to collect data, reviewed case notes and X-rays, organised and performed clinical and radiological follow-up for patients and determined reasons for non-union where possible. All data confidentiality was ensured by use of hospital number identification only and password-protected data entry. The results showed that inadequate primary fixation was the leading cause of non-union. I am currently writing this project as a paper and intend to submit it to the Journal of Foot and Ankle Surgery.*

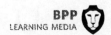

Publications

There are many ways to reference your publications, and as mentioned briefly in Chapter 3 (Application for Foundation Training) I have chosen to use, and would recommend, the Harvard style as demonstrated in the example at the end of this chapter, as it is the one with which I am most familiar. As long as it includes all of the relevant details it does not matter which format of reference you use, but remember to include your name in bold so that it is easily visible from a glance at the paper. If you have more than one publication, particularly if it is generated from a higher degree undertaken during Medical School, separate them into different sub-headings: for example 'Full manuscripts', 'Case reports', 'Published abstracts', and 'Online publications'. This shows the individual responsible for shortlisting that you have a variety of good quality publications and are aware of the literature hierarchy. If appropriate, include the PubMed Identifier number (PMID number). (Pubmed is a service of the U.S. National Library of Medicine. A unique number is assigned to all PubMed publications, which can be found by searching for your article on PubMed, though be aware that some letters and less formal publications will not have this unique identifier.) Do not under any circumstances be tempted to put your name as first author if you are not. A publication at this stage of your training is an achievement; whatever order your name comes. If it is a genuine mistake that is discovered by the selection panel it will be viewed with suspicion, and if it is discovered that you are deliberately falsifying information within your CV it could be considered a probity issue by the GMC, under the pillars of Good Medical Practice.

Presentations

When listing your presentations, again include relevant details, but you do not have to reference them as you would publications. Ensure the date, venue and the title of the presentation is included and that your name is in bold. If a fellow author presented the work you were involved in, then it is acceptable to list this here too, but make certain their name is first in the list of authors,

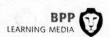

indicating them as the presenter. If you have a poster presentation, then make sure that this is clear when listing the presentation, as if it seems that you are trying to indicate a podium presentation instead, then this also looks like evidence of falsification. Use sub-headings for your presentations of 'International', 'National', 'Regional' and 'Poster' to avoid any confusion.

Scientific meetings/conferences

List any conferences or meetings you have attended in reverse chronological order with the titles, dates and places of meeting.

Teaching

If you have any formal teaching experience, including anatomy demonstration or voluntary sessions at your University post-graduation, include it within the teaching section of your CV. If you state that you have given teaching to people or groups, try to have evidence of this in the form of feedback questionnaires or Medical School evidence of involvement in student teaching. Remember, everything you put on your CV you should be able to back up at interview. As with previous chapters, the inclusion of a short statement to highlight to the shortlisters that you are aware of the needs for a doctor to have teaching skill and ability can be useful. For example:

> I have involved myself in teaching medical students and junior trainees at every stage of my career and it is an aspect of my medical career that I enjoy and recognise as important in the context of Good Medical Practice. My teaching experience includes:
>
> - Formal Anatomy volunteer teaching to medical students – Glasgow University, Dec 2008
> - Exam teaching to third-year medical students in Glasgow Royal Infirmary, Apr 2007
> - F2 Teaching Skills course – an evidence-based course for dynamic verbal and practical teaching skills. Sept 2005

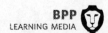

Leadership/management involvement

If you have any involvement in committees, associations or societies as a trainee, then list them here in reverse chronological order, with a brief explanation of your role. Sometimes there are things that you have been involved in that you can accidentally overlook which apply to this area, such as a member of the Hospital at Night committee, and local Clinical Governance groups or training associations that you belong to. If you have attended any formal management courses, or organised the trainee rota or teaching at any point then this is also evidence of leadership and management. Equally if you have held any positions of responsibility during Medical School, for example, captain of a sports team, head of a society, student representative, etc, then list them here also but after those that are more recent. Some medical students take part in the selection process for Medical School applicants; others are involved in the organisation of charity events or even social events like the Revue or the Graduation Ball. This is all evidence of your involvement in leadership and teamwork at all stages of your training. However, do not be tempted to fabricate, as you will always fall flat within the interview! As before, a short statement regarding your awareness of the importance of these skills is useful. For example:

> *I recognise the relevance of leadership, teamwork and management skills to training, and have involved myself in these activities at every level. My experience includes:*
>
> * *Committee Member of General Surgery Clinical Governance Group, Jan 09*
> * *General Surgery Junior Doctor Rota organiser, Western Infirmary, Apr–Aug 08*
> * *F2 Management Course – Problems Faced in Management, Oct 07*
> * *Medical Student representative for Raising and Giving Week, Nov 05*

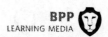

Personal interests

This section allows a bit of artistic scope. Team or individual sports are always looked upon favourably, as is evidence of seeking qualifications outside of medicine, eg SCUBA licences or foreign languages studied. If you have any outstanding achievements in these areas, then highlight it. If you have an unusual or interesting hobby, then state it; these do not have to be particularly sporty, indeed artistic hobbies can be very interesting to discuss at interview. Colleagues have been known to list 'flower-arranging' as one of their hobbies (absolutely true). Again be truthful here as there is nothing worse than stating you have a keen interest in modern art if when at interview you cannot name any artists. Do not list 'socialising with friends' and 'clubbing' for obvious reasons, even if these *are* your favourite out-of-work pastimes!

Additional experience and career intentions

This is a good section to summarise *briefly* any extra things you have done relevant to your intended specialty, ie kept a logbook of procedures/operations; completed a project or an elective in the specialty; shadowed a senior colleague in the specialty to gain additional experience; volunteered at out-of-hours GP practices; and so on. Anything that demonstrates you have shown aptitude and effort to understand and involve yourself in your future specialty will be viewed favourably by shortlisters. You should also include a key statement regarding your career intentions, but make sure to strike the right tone of confident competence in your abilities as a trainee and not arrogance. Do not be tempted into nostalgia (eg 'since childhood I have dreamed of being a radiologist...') and try not to ramble. Keep it concise, or you will lose the attention of those reviewing your CV. Try reading it out loud and see how it sounds.

Referees

If you are applying to intermediate Specialty Training you will probably be familiar with the formalities of selecting referees by

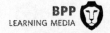

now. However, if this is your first application since graduation, these referees will be the first senior members of staff under whom you have worked in medicine. As a rule, one referee must be your current educational or clinical supervisor, but as opposed to an application form you have a degree of flexibility with regard to referees included in your CV. Having said that, it would look very odd if you didn't have a reference from anyone you had worked for over the last year! It may be preferable to choose referees allied to the specialty to which you are applying. For example, if you are applying to General Practice, you might know that Mr Surgeon will give you a very good reference and include him on the list, but it may be prudent to put Dr General Practice first. If you feel a particular person you have not worked for but you knew during Medical School will be a good referee, then by all means add them, but be aware that the shortlisters are looking for referees for whom you have worked, as they will be most qualified to comment on your skills and attributes as an employee.

Above all, when you have selected your referees, be courteous enough to ask them to act as referee before including their names. Give them plenty of notice and let them know when they are likely to be contacted. Consultants obviously see a lot of junior trainees. If they find a reference request on their desk without being asked, they are likely either to struggle to remember you, or worse, be offended that you have not been polite enough to ask. Most consultants will be grateful for a copy of your CV to peruse when writing a reference, so pre-empt this and ask them if they would like you to give them one.

Special note

The following CVs are provided as examples. The first is appropriate to a Foundation trainee applying for initial Specialty Training (ST1/CT1); the second to a trainee applying for intermediate Specialty Training (ST3). Of course, everyone has differing levels of experience; therefore there will be some overlap.

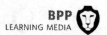

Example CV for application to initial Specialty Training

John James Smith MB CHB

Date of birth:	1 January 1984	**GMC:** 1000000
Nationality:	British	**BMA:** 200000
Address:	12 Willow Drive, Glasgow G1 1AA	**MPS:** 300000
Telephone:	0151 222 5555 / 0777333000	
E-mail:	jjsmith@doctors.org.uk	

QUALIFICATIONS

2002–2007	**University of Glasgow**	MBChB
1995–2002	**St Secondary School, London**	4 A levels

EMPLOYMENT

Future employment (Apr 09–Aug 09)	**Foundation 2 Doctor, Orthopaedic Surgery** Glasgow Royal Infirmary
Dec 08–Present	**Foundation 2 Doctor, A&E** Glasgow Royal Infirmary
Aug 08–Dec 08	**Foundation 2 Doctor, General Practice** Brookwood Practice, Glasgow
Apr 08–Aug 08	**Foundation 1 Doctor, General Surgery** Western Infirmary, Glasgow
Dec 07–Apr 08	**Foundation 1 Doctor, Paediatrics** Yorkhill Hospital, Glasgow
Aug 07–Dec 07	**Foundation 1 Doctor, General Medicine** Glasgow Royal Infirmary

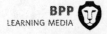

CLINICAL EXPERIENCE

My Foundation rotations have allowed me to develop and improve skills related to General Surgery. I have received positive competency-based feedback regarding my assessment, management and operative skills via structured assessment tools.

I have experience of procedures such as removal of skin lesions and have performed other surgical procedures and operations such as insertion of laparoscopic ports and abdominal closure under supervision, as evidenced by my logbook. I have shadowed senior surgeons in both elective and emergency settings to increase my knowledge and experience in this field.

COURSES

Advanced Trauma Life Support	RCS, Edinburgh	Jan 09
Generic Foundation Course	NES, Glasgow	Dec 08
Generic Foundation Course	NES, Glasgow	Oct 08
Breaking Bad News	Macmillan, Edinburgh	Apr 08
Paediatric Life Support	Resus. Council, Edinburgh	Feb 08
ILS Course	Resus. Council, Glasgow	Dec 07
A.L.E.R.T. Course	Resus. Council, Paisley	Sept 07

RESEARCH EXPERIENCE

Non-union in ankle fractures: A retrospective review. Centre of Surgical Research.

I designed and performed this retrospective study into revision surgery performed for ankle fracture non-union. Under senior guidance I performed a literature search, reviewed case notes and x-rays, organised and performed clinical and radiological follow-up for patients and determined reasons for non-union where possible. The results showed that inadequate primary fixation was the leading cause of non-union. I am currently writing this project as a paper and intend to submit it to the Journal of Foot and Ankle Surgery.

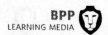

PUBLICATIONS

Letters and case reports

Smith, J. 2008. An interesting case. Journal of Medicine. 27(3), pp. 34–39.

Bloggs, J. **Smith, J.** Fellow, A. 2007. The importance of a good CV. *British Medical Journal.* 6, pp. 123–129. PMID 12848199.

PRESENTATIONS

National

The importance of a good CV. **Smith**, **J.** Bloggs, J. Fellow, A. The British CV Association Annual Meeting, London, Apr 2008.

Regional

An interesting case. **Smith, J.** Regional Audit Day Medical Directorate, Glasgow Royal Infirmary, Nov 2008.

SCIENTIFIC MEETINGS/CONFERENCES

The British CV Association Annual Meeting	Edinburgh	Apr 08
The National Trainee Surgeons Meeting	London	Jul 06

CLINICAL AUDIT

Audit of open appendicectomy. **Smith, J.** Fellow, A. Yorkhill Hospital, Glasgow, Dec 2007.

I initiated this audit which looked at the complications suffered and the length of stay associated with appendicectomy performed in our unit. I performed a literature review, identifying national guidance, collected data using a pro forma I had designed, and performed statistical analysis. Our results were compared to national standards and found to be above acceptable. The results of this audit were presented at our departmental audit meeting and a further audit is planned in a year's time to ensure we are maintaining standards and closing the audit loop.

TEACHING

I have involved myself in teaching medical students and junior trainees at every stage of my career and it is an aspect of my medical career that I enjoy

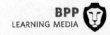

and recognise as important to Good Medical Practice. My teaching experience includes:

- Exam teaching to third-year medical students at Glasgow Royal Infirmary, Apr 2008.

- Foundation 2 Teaching Skills course – an evidence-based course for dynamic verbal and practical teaching skills, Sept 2005.

LEADERSHIP AND MANAGEMENT EXPERIENCE

I recognise the relevance of leadership, teamwork and management skills to training, and have involved myself in these activities at every level. My experience includes:

- Foundation 2 Management Course – Problems Faced in Management, Oct 2008

- Medical Student representative for Raising and Giving Week, Nov 2005

PERSONAL INTERESTS

I enjoy swimming, running and playing the acoustic guitar. I completed a half-marathon earlier this year and am currently learning French at university evening classes.

ADDITIONAL EXPERIENCE AND CAREER INTENTIONS

Since Medical School I have striven to gain experience in General Surgery. I conducted my elective in Johannesburg, South Africa in a large national hospital attending theatre and assessing patients with the trauma team for several weeks.

I have attended theatre regularly and have kept a logbook of small procedures I have performed.

It is my aim to pursue a career in General Surgery and having achieved my Foundation competencies I am confident that I can build upon this to excel as a surgical trainee.

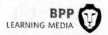

REFEREES

Mr A Consultant
Consultant General Surgeon
Canniesburn Plastic Surgery Unit
Castle Street
Glasgow
G4 0SF
Tel: 0141 111 2222 ext 1111
Email: aconsultant@ggc.nhs.uk

Miss B Consultant
Consultant Paediatric Surgeon
Yorkhill Hospital
Yorkhill Street
Glasgow
G1 000
Tel: 0141 222 3333 ext 2222
Email: bconsultant@ggc.nhs.uk

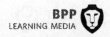

Example CV for application to intermediate Specialty Training

---

John James Smith MB CHB

Date of birth:	1 January 1982	**GMC:**	1000000
Nationality:	British	**BMA:**	200000
Address:	12 Willow Drive, Glasgow G1 1AA	**MPS:**	300000
Telephone:	0151 222 5555/0777333000		
E-mail:	jjsmith@doctors.org.uk		

QUALIFICATIONS

2008–present	**Cardiff University, Dept of Wound Healing** Multi-disciplinary distance-learning program with original research into wound healing and tissue repair	MSc
2008	**Royal College of Surgeons of England**	MRCS (A)
2000–2005	**University of Glasgow**	MBChB
1993–2000	**St Secondary School, London**	4 A levels

EMPLOYMENT

Fixed Term Specialty Training Year 2 General Surgery Rotation

Future employment (Apr 09–Aug 09)	**FTSTA2 in Colorectal Surgery** Wishaw Hospital, Lanarkshire
Dec 08–Present	**FTSTA2 in Cardiothoracic Surgery** Golden Jubilee Hospital, Glasgow
Aug 08–Dec 08	**FTSTA2 in Upper GI Surgery** Glasgow Royal Infirmary

---

Fixed Term Specialty Training Year 1 General Surgery Rotation

Apr 08–Aug 08	**FTSTA1 in General Surgery** Western Infirmary, Glasgow
Dec 07–Apr 08	**FTSTA1 in Paediatric Surgery** Yorkhill Hospital, Glasgow
Aug 07–Dec 07	**FTSTA1 in Accident and Emergency** Stobhill Hospital, Glasgow
Apr 07–Aug 07 Surgery	**Foundation 2 Doctor, Orthopaedic** Glasgow Royal Infirmary
Dec 06–Apr 07	**Foundation 2 Doctor, A&E** Glasgow Royal Infirmary
Aug 06–Dec 06	**Foundation 2 Doctor, General Practice** Brookwood Practice, Glasgow
Apr 06–Aug 06	**Foundation 1 Doctor, General Surgery** Western Infirmary, Glasgow.
Dec 05–Apr 06	**Foundation 1 Doctor, Paediatrics** Yorkhill Hospital, Glasgow
Aug 05–Dec 05	**Foundation 1 Doctor, General Medicine** Glasgow Royal Infirmary

CLINICAL EXPERIENCE

My training rotations have allowed me to develop new and enhance existing clinical, research and personal skills related to general surgery. I have over sixteen months' experience in this specialty and have received positive competency-based and multi-level feedback regarding my assessment and management of general surgical patients and operative skills via structured assessment tools.

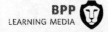

I am competent in many emergency and elective procedures such as appendicectomy, hernia repair, abscess drainage, abdominal closure and laparoscopic port insertion and manipulation. I have performed many other breast, colorectal and upper GI operations under direct supervision including mastectomy, stoma formation and cholecystectomy.

COURSES

Core Skills in Laparoscopic Surgery	RCS, London	Aug 09
Specialist Registrar Skills in Surgery	RCS, London	Jan 09
Basic Surgical Skills	RCS, Edinburgh	Nov 08
Advanced Trauma Life Support	RCS, Edinburgh	Jan 08
Generic Foundation Course	NES, Glasgow	Dec 07
Generic Foundation Course	NES, Glasgow	Oct 07
Breaking Bad News	Macmillan, Glasgow	Apr 07
A.L.E.R.T. Course	Resus. Council, Ed.	Sep 06
Paediatric Life Support	Resus. Council, Ed.	Feb 06
ILS Course	Resus. Council, Ed.	Dec 05

RESEARCH EXPERIENCE

Barrett's Oesophagus in a teenage patient. **Smith, J.** Fellow, A. Consultant, B.

This case report centred on a teenage patient presenting with severe Barrett's oesophagus after a history of several years of binge drinking. The current literature regarding the alarming trend of much younger presentation in the UK was included. This case report and review was published in the British Journal of Surgery in 2008.

Outcomes following hydradenitis surgery. **Smith, J.** Fellow, A. Consultant, B.

I designed and performed this study into the outcome measures in terms of quality of life, measured before and after excisional surgery for hydradenitis

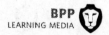

suppurativa. I appraised the literature, designed the data collection, reviewed case notes and organised and performed clinical follow-up for patients in clinic. Results showed no significant improvement in quality of life post surgery, with many patients unhappy with the scarring and recurrence rates. This study was published in the British Journal of Surgery in 2006 and I presented it at the Meeting of the Association of Surgeons of Great Britain and Ireland, 2007.

Non-union in ankle fractures: A retrospective review. **Smith, J.** Fellow, A.

I designed and performed this retrospective study into revision surgery performed for ankle fracture non-union. Under senior guidance I performed a literature search, reviewed case notes and X-rays, organised and performed clinical and radiological follow-up for patients and determined reasons for non-union where possible. The results showed that inadequate primary fixation was the leading cause of non-union. This paper was published in the British Journal of Bone and Joint Surgery in 2005.

PUBLICATIONS

Full manuscripts

Bloggs, J. **Smith, J.** Fellow, A. 2007. The importance of a good CV. British Medical Journal. 6, pp. 123–129. PMID 12848199.

Smith, J. Fellow, A. Consultant, B. 2006. Outcomes following hydradenitis surgery. BJS. 12, pp. 333–336.

Smith, J. Fellow, A. 2005. Non-union in ankle fractures: A retrospective review. BJS. 34, pp. 231–5.

Letters and case reports

Smith, J. Fellow, A. Consultant, B. 2008. Barrett's Oesophagus in a teenage patient. BJS. 8, pp. 654–9.

Smith, J. 2008. An interesting case. Journal of Medicine. 27(3), pp. 34–39.

Bloggs, J. **Smith, J.** Fellow, A. 2007. The importance of a good CV. British Medical Journal. 6, pp. 123–129. PMID 12848199.

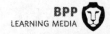

PRESENTATIONS

National

Outcomes following hydradenitis surgery. **Smith, J.** Fellow, A. Consultant, B. The Meeting of the Association of Surgeons of Great Britain and Ireland, Dec 2007.

The importance of a good CV. **Smith, J.** Bloggs, J. Fellow, A. The British CV Association Annual Meeting, London, Apr 2006.

Regional

Audit of actioning of pre-operative investigation results. **Smith, J.** Consultant, B. General Surgery Directorate Regional Audit Day. Glasgow Royal Infirmary, Apr 08.

An Interesting Case. **Smith, J.** Regional Audit Day Medical Directorate, Glasgow Royal Infirmary, Nov 2005.

SCIENTIFIC MEETINGS/CONFERENCES

The British CV Association Annual Meeting	Edinburgh	Apr 08
The Association of Surgeons of Great Britain	Belfast	Dec 07
The National Trainee Surgeons Meeting	London	Jul 05

CLINICAL AUDIT

Audit of actioning of pre-operative investigation results. **Smith, J.** Consultant, B. Glasgow Royal Infirmary, Apr 08.

This audit, which I designed, led and conducted, looked at the action taken following identification of abnormal results of investigations requested during pre-operative assessment. The results clearly indicated pathology was being missed, and led to changed management in the form of checklist identifications at different levels of the patient stay. I presented my findings at the regional audit day.

Audit of open appendicectomy. **Smith, J.** Fellow, A. Yorkhill Hospital, Glasgow, Dec 2007.

I initiated this audit, which looked at the complications suffered, and the length of stay associated with appendicectomy performed in our unit. I performed

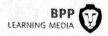

a literature review, identifying national guidance, collected data using a pro forma I had designed and performed statistical analysis. Our results were compared to national standards and found to be above acceptable. The results of this audit were presented at our departmental audit meeting and a further audit is planned in a year's time to ensure we are maintaining standards and closing the audit loop.

TEACHING

I have involved myself in teaching medical students and junior trainees at every stage of my career. It is an aspect of my medical career that I enjoy, and I recognise its importance to Good Medical Practice. My teaching experience includes:

- Formal Anatomy volunteer teaching to medical students – Glasgow University, Dec 2008.

- Exam teaching to third year medical students in Glasgow Royal Infirmary, Apr 2007.

- F2 Teaching Skills course – evidence-based course for dynamic verbal and practical teaching skills. Sept 2005.

LEADERSHIP AND MANAGEMENT EXPERIENCE

I recognise the relevance of leadership, teamwork and management skills to training, and have involved myself in these activities at every level. My experience includes:

- Committee Member of General Surgery Clinical Governance Group, Jan 09

- General Surgery Junior Doctor Rota organiser, Western Infirmary, Apr–Aug 08

- F2 Management Course – Problems Faced in Management, Oct 07

- Medical Student representative for Raising and Giving Week, Nov 05

PERSONAL INTERESTS

I enjoy swimming, running and playing the acoustic guitar. I have recently completed my first marathon, raising over £4,000 for the Macmillan charity. I continue to practice my French at university evening classes and have recently started cycling.

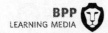

ADDITIONAL EXPERIENCE AND CAREER INTENTIONS

Since Medical School I have striven to gain experience in General Surgery. I conducted my elective in Johannesburg, South Africa in a large national hospital attending theatre and assessing patients with the trauma team for several weeks.

I have attended theatre regularly and have kept a thorough logbook of operations I have performed alone or under supervision. I have performed research and audit in General Surgery and presented and published my work. I believe I have a realistic view of a competitive, demanding specialty and have demonstrated aptitude, progression and suitability.

It is my aim to continue my Specialty Training in General Surgery and having achieved my ST1 and ST2 competencies I am confident that I can build upon my current skills and competencies to excel as an ST3 trainee.

REFEREES

Mr A Consultant
Consultant General Surgeon
Glasgow Royal Infirmary
84 Castle Street
Glasgow
G4 0SF
Tel: 0141 111 2222 ext 1111
Email: aconsultant@ggc.nhs.uk

Miss B Consultant
Consultant General Surgeon
Glasgow Royal Infirmary
84 Castle Street
Glasgow
G4 0SF
Tel: 0141 222 3333 ext 2222
Email: bconsultant@ggc.nhs.uk

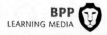

Chapter 5

Application for a Consultant Post

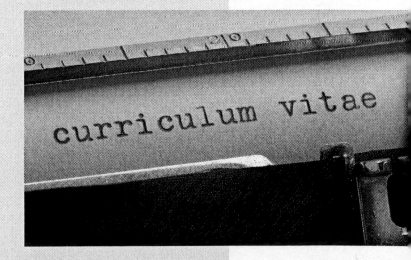

Application for a Consultant post

Introduction

By now you should have completed or nearly completed your Specialty Training and have passed any relevant fellowship exams. You will, by definition of being a senior specialty trainee, have a well-constructed CV, evidenced by the fact that you have progressed this far. However, this application is unlike any of the previous applications that you have submitted for other posts. This application is for a permanent post that you may occupy for most of your working, or indeed natural life. For this reason it is of the utmost importance that the post is right for you and that you are right for the post. Although there is increasingly scope for moving between hospitals or practices, or indeed between sub-specialty interests, you have to assume that the post you get will be the post you are still doing in ten years' time and that you will hopefully be happy to do so. Think very carefully. When applying for previous junior grade posts and even for Specialty Training there was a huge emphasis on 'getting the job' and 'getting past the hurdle', often at the cost of relocating and living wherever the jobs were available. At this final stage in your career, it is important that you and your family can feel at home living in the area.

Also consider your consultant colleagues in the department to which you are applying. These will be people you spend years working with, and you must be happy with the other personalities within the department. Ask yourself some basic questions: How do the other consultants get on? Are they cohesive or divisive as a unit? Is there one overwhelming personality who dominates the department or is it more of a team atmosphere? However important it is to you to secure a consultant position, if you address these issues earlier rather than later you can make an informed choice regarding where you apply.

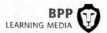

For the first time you will also need to consider the Hospital and Local Health Authority – is this a high-performing Foundation Trust or a faltering low-star hospital? What influence does the management of the hospital have here? Will they be dictating to you what you can and cannot do, and have an unhealthy influence over patient care? Or are they happy to allow the clinicians to decide on clinical priorities whilst keeping an overall eye on waiting times and national targets? This information can be gleaned by subtly questioning the other consultants in the department.

When applying for any permanent consultant position in a particular unit, you should try to include your family (if appropriate) in the decision also. Will your partner be happy in the area? How is the schooling? Where will you live relative to the hospital? How far away are other family members, and what are your plans for childcare? These issues can affect you at any stage of your career, but more junior posts are usually temporary in nature and traditionally doctors have had to commute large distances to try to address the home/work balance. This move will be permanent, and looking at these sorts of personal issues now will save trouble later.

As you can see, applying for a consultant post is a difficult decision and one where there are many more factors to appreciate than when applying at more junior grades. Ideally, you will be able to apply to a post in a hospital/practice where you have previously worked. This is good for both yourself and the department, as you will have an intimate knowledge of the dynamics of the unit and the department will know you. More importantly, they will know if they would like you to be a permanent member of the team. Most posts are eventually filled by applicants who have worked in the department previously. However, it is not always the case that the applicant will have finished their StR/SpR training within that unit – it may just be somewhere they have previously worked, even briefly, at a more junior grade earlier on in their careers, but where they flourished and parted on good relations.

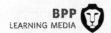

Preparation

This section of the book is laid out a little differently than the rest of the chapters, and this is because there are elements of a consultant application that do not apply to any other application, and elements of previous more junior applications are now taken for granted.

Applying for a consultant post involves a lot of preparation. You should start preparing for consultant application at least two years prior to the actual application. By years 4 (SpR) or year 6 (StR) you should be forming an idea of what part of your specialty you would most like to sub-specialise in as your future career. Unfortunately you may have to take a pragmatic view: this may not necessarily be the area of your specialty that you most enjoy. You must remember that securing a consultant post is a compromise of many different issues; for example, you may have a particular preference for a certain unit or geographical area and may decide to tailor the final stages of your training towards the experience or post availability in the unit.

If this is the case and you wish to work in a particular unit then this is the time to have an informal chat with a consultant that you get on with within the department. Ask them what it is like working in the department, and be prepared, as you may get a few interesting surprises. Consultants have many different pressures exerted upon them that junior trainees do not necessarily see. Is your friendly consultant happy working there, and do they see any problems with you working there? If all goes well and you are still happy that this is the unit you would like to work in, then make an appointment to see the Clinical Director and ask them whether they think this would be a suitable place for you to work and how you should adapt the final stages of your training to 'fill' any upcoming posts. The Clinical Director will know more than any other consultant about up-coming retrials, and any available funding for expansion. Be clear with the Clinical Director: tell them that you would be very interested in taking up a consultant post within the department and give him an

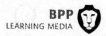

idea of the kind of sub-specialty areas you would be happy to work in – try to keep these as broad as possible, as you want to keep your options wide open. If they like you and think that you would fit well into the unit, they may even be able to delay or speed up consultant expansion to help get you on board. You need to know from them when a position is likely to come up, if they have anyone in mind for it already and what sub-specialty area it would be in.

Once you have had your discussion with the Clinical Director you need to talk to your other family members and find out what they would think of you working there and them living near there. If the sub-specialty vacancy that the unit needs to fill is not your first choice, then you need to make a decision about how much this bothers you now and how much it will bother you in the future. Above all, will you be happy doing this sub-specialty for the next few decades? Having said this, it is important to remember that practically no consultant finishes their career with the same job plan they had at the start.

In summary the decision to apply for a consultant post must not be taken lightly. You must feel that you are ready to do the job and all that it entails. This means that you must overcome one or two last hurdles. First, you need to gain sufficient clinical experience to perform at an adequate and competent level in all areas of your consultant practice. Second, if you are in a surgical specialty, you must pass your final exit exam and in this case the two hurdles are often linked.

Fellowships

Fellowships are normal practice in many specialties, although in a small number they are almost unheard of. There are two types of fellowship that most doctors apply for. The first type is for a prolonged period of time, usually six to twelve months, where a trainee works in a different unit to improve their clinical skills, possibly undertake some research, experience the specialist interests of another unit and generally broaden their horizons

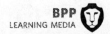

both personally and professionally. These fellowships can be in the UK or abroad, which is also a consideration if you have a family here. However, if it is feasible, time living abroad with your family on a fellowship can be very enjoyable and a perk rather than a drawback of the training process.

The second type of fellowship is where a trainee visits a number of different units to gain experience of certain techniques or institutions. These tend to be shorter visits, where the trainee is there primarily as an observer, and can last up to three months. In most cases these three months can be counted as Out Of Programme Experience (OOPE) and should not affect the date of your completion of training. However, this needs to be agreed in advance with your Dean and the Postgraduate Medical Education and Training Board (PMETB) or equivalent.

It is highly advisable to go on some sort of fellowship as it shows determination, distinguishes you from the other applicants and demonstrates commitment to a particular sub-specialty area (hopefully one where you know there is an upcoming post in a place you would like to work!). You should research institutions and individuals well in advance and find somewhere you would like to visit. Try to speak to someone who has visited there previously as they may give you some pointers or even an introduction.

Applications for fellowships tend to be fairly informal and an email to the head of the relevant department, with a copy of your CV attached should generally suffice. If one of your consultants knows the head of department personally, then it may be wise to ask them if they would be willing to send an email or letter of support for your fellowship application. In terms of your CV, it is normally possible to simply update the one you used for securing your Specialty Training position with any additional publications and presentations. Be sure to state in an 'Objectives' section on the front page of the CV why you feel visiting and/ or working in this department would aid your development as a clinician (see the example at the end of this chapter).

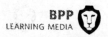

If appropriate, you also need to decide when is best to sit your exit exam and I would recommend doing this early enough that you have a couple of sittings available prior to going away on your fellowship. You will feel much more confident and comfortable as a visiting trainee if you have this hurdle out of the way prior to going and working elsewhere. You will also then be able to devote all your time and energy to picking up the vital clinical experience that you need to become a consultant.

The application process

By this stage you will be completing your training, having finished all your relevant exams, and hopefully you will have been on a fellowship. You now should be in a position to apply for a consultant post. If you do not feel that you are ready to take up a consultant position at this stage in your training, then you might want to consider asking the postgraduate Dean for permission for a 'period of grace', which extends your training for a maximum of six months. The alternative option is to consider applying for a 'post completion of training' fellowship to enhance your clinical skills further.

Hopefully you will now feel able to apply for a consultant post, which you can do if the interview dates for the post are within three months of the date of your completion of training. In many cases there may be a time period during which you are waiting for the job you are interested in applying for to be released. If this is the case, it may be worthwhile contacting your Postgraduate Dean early to apply for that 'period of grace', so that if you have a few more months to wait before the job comes out, you can continue in your current post, thereby avoiding clinical de-skilling and being unemployed.

Hopefully the consultant position now being advertised is the one from the department you visited a couple of years ago, and is in the sub-specialty area you are expecting to perform. In preparing well for this moment, you will have undertaken the appropriate type of sub-specialty fellowship and can feel

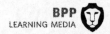

reassured that due to your previous conversations with your friendly consultant and the Clinical Director, the department know you are applying for the position and are happy for you to do so.

The stories of posts being advertised where the candidate has written the person specification and is the only applicant are all but myth. Don't be afraid to find that a number of people have applied and if you are not the internal candidate, be aware that there may be one. Whilst it is sometimes believed that the vast majority of appointments are all but decided prior to the interview, it is a fact that if there are two very closely matched candidates with differing supporters and one performs badly in interview and the other performs well, then it stands to reason that it is almost always the candidate who performs well who will get the job. However, if you have had no experience of the unit, haven't done the right fellowships and don't have a strong CV it doesn't matter how well you perform at interview – the fact of the matter is that you are not going to secure that post.

The person specification and tailoring your CV

Job adverts for consultant positions are very detailed and must, according to NHS policy, include a variety of information. They should include information about the specifics of the post, the department, the hospital and usually some information about the geographical area. The advert should state whether this is a new post or a replacement. This is important; if it is a replacement, you will be inheriting somebody else's patients. The advert should state a suggested job plan, subject to agreement with the applicant appointed, and a person specification. The person specifications are particularly important, as they give you information that you must include in your application. You must go through the list of essential criteria and make sure you have, or fulfil, them all. You should go down the desirable criteria and make sure there is a clear reference to these criteria within your CV. For example, if a desirable criterion is experience of a particular technique, and you have done this during your fellowship, then

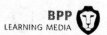

make absolutely sure that this is clearly mentioned in your CV, to increase the chances of being shortlisted.

During your medical career you will have picked up the majority of essentials that you require on your CV. If you didn't already have these, you would not be in the position you are now. These essentials include clinical audits, research, presentations, and publications. However, there are a couple of extra fields, listed below, that tend to be more important when applying for a consultant position and these are often found in the 'desirable' section of the person specification criteria and require some preparation.

Management experience

Any conversation with any Clinical Director of any specialty will inform you of how important it is to function effectively as a manager as well as a doctor. Evidence that you have tried to achieve this before your consultant applications shows foresight, vision and preparation – all of which are good qualities in doctors or managers. Therefore, if you have not done so already, you should book and attend some form of management course. This should be done well in advance of your application. Courses exist, and are organised into several days in a single block of study or several days over a period of time. Check with your own postgraduate medical education centre or Deanery as they may offer some suitable courses. These courses are often split into management sub-type areas, such as leadership, time management, problems in management and people skills, and may cover areas such as recruitment and retention, medico-legal issues and dealing with conflict and complaints – all of which will look great on your CV.

Teaching experience

Another area which tends to appear on the Consultant person specification is attendance at some sort of formal teaching course. As a Consultant, you will be directly responsible for teaching and training, which as you know is one of the pillars of Good

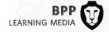

Medical Practice. Therefore, if the last time you attended one of these courses was when you were a junior doctor, it is probably wise to attend another one now that you are so much more advanced in your career. Evidence of your efforts to improve your skills in these areas will be looked upon favourably. You can book yourself on to these courses in similar ways to the management courses, but they may also be advertised at the beginning of publications such as *BMJ Careers*.

 ## Key preparation points

- Prepare as early as possible. Start formulating a plan at least two years prior to application
- Approach units you may wish to work in early
- Remember to consider whether you will enjoy living and working in the area
- Think about the timing of fellowships and, if appropriate, exams
- If you are planning a fellowship, inform the Deanery early
- Improve the Management section of your CV
- Attend a teaching skills course

 ## Key CV construction points

- Always present information in reverse chronological order (most recent first)
- Avoid fancy fonts: ease of reading is the aim! Arial, Calibri and Cambria are personal favourites, but any font that is clear and easy to read is unlikely to offend
- Font size: no smaller than ten, twelve if possible. A shortlister that is reading dozens of CVs is likely to be irritated if having to squint
- Paragraphs: to save space, do not start a new paragraph unnecessarily
- Spacing: you will extend the length of your CV if you double-space everything. A ten-page CV is unnecessary when a four-page version would suffice
- 'I': avoid the use of the word 'I' as it can become very repetitive
- Length: historically the 'keep to two pages' rule has been applied. Less than five and more than one is recommended
- Alignment: try to keep everything symmetrical, consistent and in alignment. There are fancy computer programs that can do this for

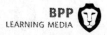

you, but a keen eye, printing out a test copy and looking at it carefully will achieve the same result

- Bold and underlining: avoid overuse. Employ headings to highlight areas of importance and use the bold function sparingly, eg for your surname on any publications. Do not be tempted to mix and match these throughout your CV, as it will cause confusion. Stick to one
- Bullet points can be very useful to summarise information clearly and succinctly but do not overuse them
- Acronyms: as individuals responsible for shortlisting may be from a different specialty, avoid the use of acronyms

Writing the CV

A CV for a consultant application is aiming to give a slightly more polished and mature appearance than your previous CVs, and some of the sections which were previously included and had much focus, eg clinical audit, become less important as they are assumed by your higher level of experience. In that vein, other sections increase in importance such as teaching and management. Above all clarity is key; therefore you will have to consider culling parts of your CV to ensure you maintain its clarity.

Personal/professional details

Include your full name, address and telephone numbers (at least work and mobile) as well as your GMC number, National Training Number (NTN), BMA number if appropriate and Medical Indemnity Membership number. As with previous chapters, for ease of reading and conservation of space, keep your contact and personal details on the left and your professional details on the right (see the example at the end of this chapter).

Objectives

Immediately following the Personal details section, it is good to have a succinct summary of exactly what stage you are at in your career and what your intentions are. You should aim to comment upon your preferred sub-specialty interests at this

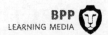

stage but keep this part short and punchy. Make sure to strike the right tone of confident competence in your abilities and not arrogance. This can be achieved by listing your areas of interest and competence and then highlighting the skills you wish to continue to develop (for example on your fellowships).

Sub-specialty experience/fellowships

You must look carefully at the person specification for the position you are applying for, and tailor this section extremely carefully to what is written. If the person specification is asking for a candidate with experience in two or three sub-specialty areas, then make sure that you have these, that you list them here and that for each one you explain what experience you have and where you gained it. You might want to comment on which consultants in the sub-specialty areas you have worked with. Hopefully, these sub-specialty areas will relate to the fellowships you have completed, and under the sub-specialty headings you can comment on the experience you gained in these areas during your fellowships.

Qualifications and prizes/distinctions

Always include the university/professional body where your qualifications were gained and the dates. It is probably no longer valuable to list your A level results, especially as if you are currently eligible to be applying for consultant positions it is possible that your results will seem poor in relation to modern pass rates!

Employment

List your current employment first; followed by your previous jobs with the inclusive grade, specialty and hospital in reverse chronological order, with the most recent first. At this stage of your applications, when this section is likely to be very long, it is worth considering having your previous posts split into ordered sections, the titles of which will depend on whether you trained during the older SpR system or the newer Foundation/

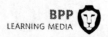

Specialty Training system. The exemplar CV given at the end of the chapter will display the newer system, but for example if you are a Plastic Surgery trainee who completed a Basic Surgical Training programme, then a Higher Surgical Training programme, you can list it as follows:

West of Scotland Higher Surgical Training General Surgery Rotation

Aug 05–Present	**Specialist Registrar, Plastic surgery**	Glasgow Royal Infirmary

West of Scotland Basic Surgical Training Programme

Feb 05–Aug 05	**SHO in Plastic Surgery**	Glasgow Royal Infirmary
Aug 04–Feb 05	**SHO in Orthopaedics**	Wishaw Hospital, Lanarkshire
Feb 04–Aug 04	**SHO in Urology**	Western Infirmary, Glasgow
Aug 03–Feb 04	**SHO in Paediatric**	Yorkhill Hospital, Glasgow
Feb 03–Aug 03	**SHO in General Surgery**	Monklands Hospital, Lanarkshire
Aug 02–Feb 03	**SHO in ENT Surgery**	Gartnaval Hospital, Glasgow

---

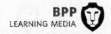

Courses

List all completed courses with their dates (in reverse chronological order as always) and also the location and course provider, eg Royal College of Surgeons for ATLS and the Resuscitation Council for ALS.

Clinical experience

At this stage of your training, this section can now be a brief explanation of your years of experience in your specialty, with particular reference to any specialist procedures that you can perform. Do not simply list parts of your logbook. Remember your logbook is now assessed through the system of annual review and also by the Postgraduate Medical Education and Training Board (PMETB) when issuing your Completion of Training certificate, which you need to produce to start any position at consultant level.

Clinical audit

At this stage in your training the Clinical audit section should be emphasised less on your CV. You should have a few examples listed of audits you have completed, and hopefully at this stage, supervised. You should also include any titles of audits that you are currently performing, or preferably supervising.

Research experience

If you have completed a research degree then list the thesis title, university at which it was examined and dates. Include a succinct explanation of your research and what this led to in terms of publications, presentations and award of a further degree.

Publications

Hopefully by now this section will have a lot of material. As mentioned in previous chapters, there are many ways to reference your publications, the Harvard style is shown in the example below, but any style that you are familiar with is acceptable.

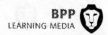

Ensure your surname is in bold so that it is easily visible from a glance at the CV. To display your publications in a clear and logical fashion, separate them into the sub-headings such as 'Full manuscripts', 'Case reports', 'Published abstracts', and 'Online publications'. At this stage I hardly need mention that you should take care to ensure your surname is in the correct position in the author list, as if it is not and this is perceived as an attempt to falsify your CV, the implications are grave.

Presentations

List your presentations clearly and logically, again separating them into International, National, etc. Ensure your name is in bold and the date, venue and the title of the presentation is included. If a fellow author presented the work you were involved in, then it is acceptable to list this here too, but make certain their name is first in the list of authors, indicating them as the presenter.

Meetings attended

List all scientific meetings attended with the dates and venues in reverse chronological order.

Teaching

Make reference here to any teaching you have delivered or training courses you have taught on or organised. If you have any experience of delivering teaching or giving lectures in the university then explain this here, especially if you were given formal instruction on teaching techniques such as facilitator training. If you have managed to do a formal teaching course then list this here also.

Leadership/management involvement

This is an important section when applying for a consultant post, and you should have completed a management course of some sort by this stage. If this course is modular, be sure to

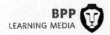

give the titles of the modules you have attended. If you have any leadership roles, past or present, for example if you are a representative for any associations, committees or societies then include then here.

Personal interests

The 'Interests' section will probably follow the same format as your previous CVs'. Include any outstanding extra-curricular achievements, foreign languages studied or hobbies pursued. Again it is prudent to be truthful here. Remember that the interviewers may know you quite well!

Referees

You should aim to have a minimum of three consultant referees, the first of whom should be from your current unit. Make sure you approach these individuals early and give them a copy of your CV, otherwise they will struggle when writing your reference.

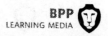

Example CV for application to a Consultant post

John James Smith MBCHB MRCS MD

Date of birth:	1st January 1978	**GMC:**	1000000
Nationality:	British **BMA:**	200000	
Address:	12 Willow Drive, Glasgow G1 1AA	**MPS:**	300000 NTN: WOS/ K6/003/N
Telephone:	0151 222 5555/0777333000		
E-mail:	jjsmith@doctors.org.uk		

OBJECTIVES

I am a Specialist Registrar at Famous Plastic Surgery Unit, Glasgow Royal Infirmary, and I am due to complete training in February 2010. My areas of sub-specialty interest are burns surgery, lower limb trauma and breast reconstruction. I intend to visit St. Excellent Hospital in Texas, Professor J Bloggs in Boston and Professor J Doe in Canada between October and December 2009. These are leading burns surgery units and I intend to learn new techniques and skills that I can bring back to Glasgow.

BURNS SURGERY EXPERIENCE

I have extensive previous Burns Surgery experience and was employed as a Burns Surgery Fellow between August 2002 and August 2003, during which time I performed 1,400 burns surgery cases. I have extensive experience of managing paediatric burns gained whilst working at the Sick Children's Hospital.

I have conducted research in Burns Surgery comparing different modalities to measure early burn depth. This has led to three first-author full manuscript publications and nine oral presentations and two posters at international and national meetings. My research has led to the award of my MD from Glasgow University.

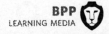

LOWER LIMB TRAUMA EXPERIENCE

I have extensive experience of complex lower limb trauma and was employed as Trauma Fellow between August 2003 and August 2004. I have performed over 65 free flap tissue transfers for the reconstruction of lower leg soft tissue defects, and in 22 of these I was the lead surgeon, responsible for the planning and performance of these procedures with little or no consultant input. The majority of these flaps were anterior lateral thigh flaps and free latissimus dorsi flaps. I have previously taught on the combined Orthopaedic and Plastic surgery 'Lower limb Trauma' Course and the Plastic Surgery 'Flap Course', teaching candidates how to debride, skin graft and raise free flaps. I have also tutored on the Microsurgery course for trainees, demonstrating vascular and neural anastomoses.

I have been taught techniques in free tissue transfer by many consultants, including Mr A Famous, Miss B Renowned, Mr C Prestigious and Miss D Revered.

QUALIFICATIONS

2002–2004	University of Glasgow	MD
2002	Royal College of Surgeons of England	MRCS
1995–2000	University of Glasgow	MBChB
1990–1995	St Secondary School, London	

EMPLOYMENT

Pan-Scotland Specialist Training Programme in Plastic Surgery

Aug 07–Present   **Specialist Registrar, Plastic Surgery**
Glasgow Royal Infirmary

Aug 04–Aug 07   **Specialist Registrar, Plastic Surgery**
Aberdeen Royal Infirmary

Aug 03–Aug 04   **Trauma Fellow, Plastic Surgery**
Glasgow Royal Infirmary

Aug 02–Aug 03   **Burns Fellow, Plastic Surgery**
Glasgow Royal Infirmary

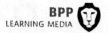

West of Scotland Foundation Training Programme

Apr 02–Aug 02	**SHO, Plastic Surgery** Glasgow Royal Infirmary
Dec 01–Apr 02	**SHO, Orthopaedic Surgery** Western Infirmary, Glasgow
Aug 01–Dec 01	**SHO, A&E Medicine** Stobhill Hospital, Glasgow
Apr 01–Aug 01	**House Officer, General Surgery** Wishaw Hospital, Lanarkshire
Dec 00–Apr 01	**House Officer, General Medicine** Ayr Hospital, Ayrshire
Aug 00–Dec 00	**House Officer, Plastic Surgery** Glasgow Royal Infirmary

CLINICAL EXPERIENCE

I have over seven years of Plastic Surgery experience and have trained in Glasgow and Aberdeen. I have performed a wide range of elective and emergency cases as the lead surgeon including many free tissue transfers, as evidenced by my logbook. I have extensive experience in both trauma and burns cases and have performed research into burn depth measurement. I have published my work in peer-reviewed journals and presented at international and national meetings.

COURSES

Doctor as Manager	NES, Glasgow	May 09
Teaching the Teachers	NES, Glasgow	Jan 08
Advanced Hand Surgery	RCS, London	Nov 07
Advanced Trauma Life	RCS, Edinburgh	Apr 06
Care of the Critically Ill Surgical Patient	RCS, Glasgow	Nov 05
Microsurgical Skills	Northwick Park, London	Nov 02

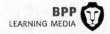

| Basic Surgical Skills | RCS, Leicester | Jun 02 |
| Advanced Life Support | Resus. Council, Edinburgh | Feb 02 |

RESEARCH EXPERIENCE

MD Thesis: The early investigation of paediatric burn depth

MD awarded from Glasgow University Medical School November 2004

My thesis explores the reliability and validity of measurement of early burn depth (within the first seventy-two hours of injury) using invasive and non-invasive methods. These methods are compared in several projects with differing variables, points explored. My research led to three first-author publications and eight presentations at international and national meetings.

PUBLICATIONS

Full manuscripts

Smith, J. Bloggs, J. Fellow, A. 2007. Even more measurement of early burn depth with Laser Doppler imaging and Histology. Burns. 111, pp. 111–222. PMID 12848112.

Smith, J. Bloggs, J. Fellow, A. 2006. More measurement of early burn depth with Laser Doppler imaging and Histology. Burns. 222, pp. 111–222. PMID 12848199.

Smith, J. Bloggs, J. Fellow, A. 2005. Measurement of early burn depth with Laser Doppler imaging and Histology. Burns. 333, pp. 111–222. PMID 12848110.

Smith, J. Bloggs, J. Fellow, A. 2004. Principles of measurement of early burn depth with Laser Doppler imaging and Histology. Burns. 444, pp. 111–222. PMID 12848111.

Online publications

Smith, J. 2006. Some interesting facts. *Society of Medicine*. www.societyofmedicine/jbloggs.com

Letters and case reports

Smith, J. 2007. Another interesting case. *Journal of Medicine*. 27(3), pp. 34–39.

Smith, J. 2002. An interesting case. *Journal of Medicine*. 17(3), pp. 35–43.

BPP
LEARNING MEDIA

Published abstracts

Smith, J. 2001. Facts about an interesting case. *Journal of Medicine*. 27(3), pp. 34–39.

PRESENTATIONS

International

Final Measurement of early burn depth with Laser Doppler imaging and Histology. **Smith, J.** Bloggs, J. Fellow, A. The International Burns Meeting, Texas, July 2006.

Further Measurement of early burn depth with Laser Doppler imaging and Histology. **Smith, J.** Bloggs, J. Fellow, A. Another International Burns Meeting, Istanbul, Jan 2005.

Measurement of early burn depth with Laser Doppler imaging and Histology. **Smith, J.** Bloggs, J. Fellow, A. Yet Another International Burns Meeting, Zurich, June 2004.

National

More burns presentations. **Smith, J.** Bloggs, J. Fellow, A. The National Burns Meeting, Belfast, April 2006.

Another burns presentation. **Smith, J.** Bloggs, J. Fellow, A. The National Burns Meeting, London, July 2003.

An interesting case. **Smith, J.** National Plastic Surgery Meeting, Glasgow, Nov 2004.

SCIENTIFIC MEETINGS/CONFERENCES

The British Association of Plastic and Reconstructive Surgeons	London	Jul 09
The British Association of Plastic and Reconstructive Surgeons	Bristol	Dec 08
Yet Another International Burns Meeting	Texas	Jul 06
Another International Burns Meeting	Belfast	Apr 06

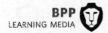

The International Burns Meeting	Istanbul	Jan 05
Another National Burns Meeting	Zurich	Jun 04
The National Burns Meeting	London	Jul 03
The British Association of Plastic and Reconstructive Surgeons	London	Dec 02

CLINICAL AUDIT

Current

Audit of nipple necrosis in breast reductions (Supervising junior colleague).

Past

Audit of abdominoplasty complications. Fellow, A, **Smith, J.** Glasgow Royal Infirmary, Dec 2007.

Audit of free flap failures. **Smith, J.** Senior, A. Aberdeen Royal Infirmary. 2006 (Presented at BAPRAS 2007).

Audit of tendon ruptures. Colleague, B, **Smith, J.** Glasgow Royal Infirmary, June 2005 (Published in Annals of Plastic Surgery).

TEACHING

- Organiser and teacher on Lower limb Trauma and Free Flap Courses, Glasgow 2006–2009.

- Tutor on Microsurgery course for trainees, Glasgow 2005–2009.

- Teaching the Teachers formal teaching course completed – Jan 2008.

- Teacher on Plastic Surgery SHO Teaching Programme 2004–2006.

LEADERSHIP/MANAGEMENT EXPERIENCE

- 'Doctor as Manager' Management Course   May 2009

- Representative, Scottish Plastic Surgery Training Association   2008–2009

- Committee Member, Association of Surgeons in Training   2006–2008

- President, Plastic Surgery Trainees Association   2005–2006

PERSONAL INTERESTS

I enjoy swimming, running and playing tennis. I completed a half-marathon earlier this year and am currently training for my first marathon.

REFEREES

Mr A Consultant
Consultant Plastic Surgeon
Canniesburn Plastic Surgery Unit

Glasgow Royal Infirmary
84 Castle Street
Glasgow
G4 0SF
Tel: 0141 111 2222 ext 1111
Email: aconsultant@ggc.nhs.uk

Miss B Consultant
Consultant Plastic Surgeon
Canniesburn Plastic Surgery Unit

Glasgow Royal Infirmary
84 Castle Street
Glasgow
G4 0SF
Tel: 0141 222 3333 ext 2222
Email: bconsultant@ggc.nhs.uk

Mr C Consultant
Consultant Plastic Surgeon
Plastic Surgery Unit
Aberdeen Royal Infirmary
Forester Hill
Aberdeen,
AB25 2ZN
Tel: 0845 111 2222 ext 3333
Email: cconsultant@ari.nhs.uk

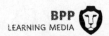

Chapter 6

Application forms

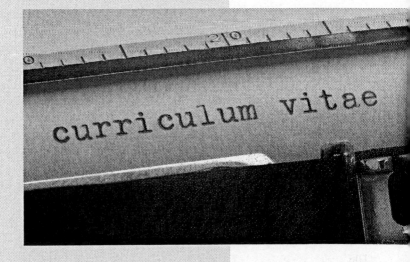

Application forms

Introduction

As this book concentrates on the construction of the medical CV, this chapter will not delve too deeply into the process of filling in applications forms. The reason for this is that application forms, although increasingly more generic across the specialties, are constantly changing in composition year after year, making it difficult to generalise a structured template. However, the majority of application forms are based on a more ordered version of a CV, and much of the information is repeated.

Recently, application forms have added in more abstract questions that are there to test the insight and commitment of the candidate to the specialty, with specific marks assigned for this. Many of the application forms released by deaneries, usually via a website, also have a guidance document attached. You should read this, as even if the majority of the form is relatively self-explanatory, there will often be small formatting guidance or techniques they would prefer you to use when answering questions (see STAR later in this chapter) and losing vital marks due to carelessness is not desirable.

We reviewed a selection of surgical specialty application forms at the end of the 2008 application process to see if there emerged a pattern or theme amongst the forms regarding the type of question posed and evidence required to gain points. We compared this with our medical colleagues and found a similar trend. The usual headings covered in the CV were there as always, covering your qualifications, prizes and distinctions, courses attended, experience of audit/research/teaching, etc, but as the form progressed more lateral questions emerged. Themes became apparent from our review, the most common of which are explored below. It is by no means an exhaustive list but should give you some guidance as to the type of questions likely to be asked and the sort of evidence that could be provided. Please remember, this is not specific to any particular level of training

BPP
LEARNING MEDIA

and must be tailored to your own experience and position. Examples are provided where possible, but these are for structure and guidance and your own answers must obviously be drawn from your own personal experiences.

Undergraduate and postgraduate achievements

A common question to ask is to detail your undergraduate or postgraduate achievements. There is usually a specific section for prizes and distinctions, but if not, or the award does not fit specifically into this category, then detail it here. Good areas to focus on are your elective or special study modules and any distinctions or particular clinical experience you gained from these. If you studied a foreign language and attained any formal grade, then this ceases to be an interest and becomes an achievement. This section is mainly for academic or academically related subjects, with sporting or other achievements usually reserved for the 'Other achievements' section.

Current post

A common question is to ask you to describe the duties you perform in your current post. This can give the individuals shortlisting a chance to see the level of responsibility of your current role, the clinical areas that you cover and the on-call duties you perform. Do not forget to include some form of reference to your clinical governance activities like audit, teaching, morbidity and mortality. For example:

> As a Foundation 2 doctor on the Cardiology team, my commitments are split between acute medical on-calls, ward cover and elective clinic and cardiac procedure sessions.
> My elective duties involve attending daily ward rounds, assisting the Foundation 1 doctor, and attending my consultants' cardiac procedure sessions and clinics.
>
> When second on call for medicine I take acute referrals from A&E and regional hospitals, assess all new ward referrals and

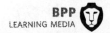

cover the medical admissions unit. Organisation of the daily acute medical handovers and co-ordination of other specialty referrals are also my responsibility.

I attend monthly Cardiology audit meetings, Morbidity and Mortality meetings and Medical Grand Rounds, at which I have presented my clinical audit. I attend regional Foundation and departmental Cardiology teaching.

Clinical competencies

A common question in all the application forms reviewed was to describe current competencies in relation to the specialty applied for. These types of questions can be quite difficult to answer as they can appear vague. Competencies can encompass many things to do with procedures, clinical skills, research and management. If it is clearly stated under a heading of 'Clinical/procedural competencies', then depending on the word count allowed, or space in the text box, try to be logical and list your skills as appropriate to your level of experience. For example, an applicant for Orthopaedic Specialist Training may put:

I am competent in the assessment and emergency management of simple and open fractures including those involving tissue loss, dislocated joints and septic arthritis. I hold a valid ATLS certificate and am experienced in the safe assessment and management of varied trauma. I maintain awareness of my limitations and when to involve more experienced colleagues, for example in the definitive management of compound lower limb trauma and complex hand injury.

My elective orthopaedic skills include removal of metalwork, assisting in joint arthroplasty and tendon reconstruction. I have broad experience in the assessment and management of the seriously ill surgical patient and am experienced in multi-disciplinary teamworking, having passed CCRISP and ALS.

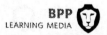

Listed below are the numbers of common operations I have performed independently or under direct supervision

- *Manipulation of closed fractures – 22*
- *Washout/debridement of wounds – 18*
- *Extensor tendon repair – 9*
- *Hip hemiarthroplasty – 3*
- *Total hip replacement – 2*

If the question is not as clearly defined, and there is space available, it may be worth adding further headings, such as 'Research competencies' and 'Management competencies'. For example:

Research competencies

I am experienced in the design, initiation and process of research projects and case reports, have published in peer-reviewed journals and presented at national meetings.

I have a wide experience of conducting clinical audit, including re-audit, closure of the audit loop and the presentation and publication of my work.

I keep up to date with current literature in orthopaedic surgery and have attended national meetings, most recently The British Elbow and Shoulder Society, 2010.

Management competencies

'Management for Doctors' – Management course for senior medical trainees 2008.

Junior Doctor rota organisation in Birmingham 2007.

Head of Surgical Society, Birmingham Medical School 2003–2004.

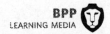

Clinical audit/research

In application forms, you will either be asked to list the audits or research projects you have been involved in, usually with a small summary of your role (just like the CV), or to choose ONE audit or research project that is particularly relevant and describe how it changed practice. Read the form carefully: if they are asking for your personal involvement, do not choose a study that scientifically was very impressive, but in which you were not significantly involved and are listed as fourth author. Equally, it is more relevant to give an example of something recent (ie last two years) that has been shown to alter or reassess clinical practice at your unit.

As mentioned, many deaneries will produce guidance documents, which aim to help the candidate to fill in these forms, therefore do not ignore them! Most of them prefer the STAR method of answering these questions, where you describe a Situation you were involved in or Task you were set; the Action that you took (explaining why), and the Result of your action. This has to be related back to the question asked. For example:

I noticed that there had been a recent increase in the complications suffered by patients at our unit who had undergone appendicectomy. After discussion with my consultant, I initiated an audit, which examined the complications suffered and the length of stay associated with appendicectomy performed in our unit on all patients over the previous six months. I performed a literature review, identifying national guidance regarding complication rates and length of hospital stay associated with appendicectomy, and using a pro forma I had designed I collected anonymous retrospective data from patients' case notes. I analysed the results statistically and found that when compared to national standards, our results were above acceptable. The results of this audit were presented at our departmental audit meeting and a further audit is planned in a year's time to ensure we are maintaining these standards and to close the audit loop.

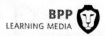

This clearly follows the STAR guidance. The Situation/Task was the identification of a recent surge in complications and the raised concern. The Action was the initiation and conduct of the audit. The Result was the good departmental results, which were shared at the department meeting and the planning of a further audit. The other thing to notice is that by explaining the steps in this manner; you are letting the shortlisters know that you are aware of the steps associated with clinical audit/research and your personal involvement with every stage.

Communication skills

Many generic application forms include sections pertaining to communication skills, and ask you to provide an example of a situation where you have displayed these skills. This is hard to do, particularly as there can be a stringent word count. I would advise drawing from real experience, as making up a situation will not only be difficult to describe if you are invited for interview, but false situations tend to be over-embellished when written and come across as untrue on the forms. These situations need not be heroic or glamorous, just displaying everyday communication with patients, relatives or colleagues. Although they do not need to be medically orientated, often the best examples are work-related. Think of a situation where you were pleased with your communication, for example a sensitively broken piece of bad news, a misunderstanding that you resolved or a colleague-related tension that you handled well. Again follow the STAR approach of answering such questions: Situation, Task, Action, Result. For example:

> *I was recently involved in a case where a paediatric patient had unfortunately had their operation cancelled after starving all morning due to an emergency trauma that had overrun. The patient's parents were furious, abusive to the nursing staff and were demanding to see the consultant, who was in theatre operating on the trauma case. I explained by taking them through the procedure of our booking system for trauma that such accidents were unpredictable and unfortunately resulted*

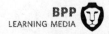

in the occasional elective cancellation. I apologised for their understandable distress, assured them that the consultant would come to see them after the emergency operation and offered myself as a point of contact if they needed further information. They were satisfied with my explanation and mentioned to my consultant when she saw them how helpful it had been to have the reason for the cancellation and the booking system explained by a member of the team.

By explaining the entire scenario in the STAR manner, you can highlight the areas where you displayed good and effective communication, and then round up nicely at the end with a statement regarding the feedback received regarding your communication.

Initiative

A question that is sometimes asked by application forms is how you can demonstrate where you have shown initiative in a situation. This is very vague, and again is not restricted to medicine. Try to think of a time where through your own ingenuity you have come up with an idea or plan that has changed something for the better. Have you redesigned a rota? Have you implemented a teaching programme? Did you change the way Raising and Giving week was conducted at your Medical School? Only use examples from the past two years, otherwise it seems as if these areas of good practice in which you have previously excelled have now been neglected. There is more scope for artistic license here. Again, follow the STAR pattern and show the individuals shortlisting that you have a spark. For example, a Foundation applicant might put:

During my final year at university I became aware that the two-hour 'Campus Tour' to show prospective undergraduates around our university and to answer any questions was poorly attended by current final-year medical students, as it coincided with one of the busiest revision periods of the year. As ambassadors for our Medical School, I felt it important to give prospective

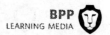

undergraduates a good welcome by a range of students from all years to answer any questions. I therefore organised a rota amongst my year where we could take turns at the tour, swapping at hourly intervals so that all participants would only have an hour away from their study groups. This format was so well received by students and prospective undergraduates that it was adopted formally by the Medical Education Department and continued.

If there is any hard evidence of the examples that you give in these questions, (and unfortunately, due to the nature of them, this is often not the case) then make some reference to it at the end of the answer. For example at the end of the above example:

This format was so well received by students and prospective undergraduates that it was adopted formally by the Medical Education Department and continued, and I received a thank you letter from the undergraduate admissions tutor.

Issues related to clinical governance and risk management

Some forms will ask you to outline an event you were involved in where issues relating to clinical governance or risk management were raised. The most important thing to do before attempting a question like this is to consider your definitions of these terms. The Department of Health, General Medical Council and British Medical Journal websites are good places to start. It is not as intimidating a concept as it sounds. The Department of Health defines clinical governance as:

A system through which NHS organisations are accountable for continuously improving the quality of their services and safeguarding high standards of care, by creating an environment in which clinical excellence will flourish.

(Department of Health website, 2009)

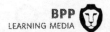

The six pillars of clinical governance are:

1. Clinical effectiveness
2. Research & development
3. Openness
4. Risk management
5. Education & training
6. Clinical audit

This means that anything related to these topics is really a clinical governance issue, therefore your answers have a large degree of scope. You could easily use the clinical audit example earlier in this chapter as evidence of clinical governance experience, as an area of potentially increased complications had been noticed and an audit initiated to investigate. Another example could be:

> *Upon commencing a recent position, it came to my attention that no departmental junior doctor teaching programme existed. As the regional teaching programme is held at another hospital, many colleagues who were on nights, covering wards or on call, were missing this vital part of education and training. Identifying this as a clinical governance issue, I raised it with my Educational Supervisor, who had not been aware of the situation and supported me in the initiation of junior doctor-led teaching, supervised by a nominated consultant each week. This meant that though we were responsible for our own learning, we were in a facilitated and supported environment, resulting in improved specialty knowledge, morale and departmental relations.*

Risk management, as a pillar of clinical governance, is a uniform process set in place to reduce errors, accidents and injury to NHS patients and staff and to improve safety and quality. It can focus on risk to the individual (ie patient/staff member), risk to the trust (litigation) and risk to the organisation (NHS reputation). Areas that are included in this are drug errors, health and safety at work, immunisations, needle-stick injuries and MRSA, for example.

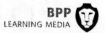

Identification and analysis of risk is the subject of a separate book, but questions regarding it are looking for you to display knowledge of what risk management involves and your understanding of how it is identified and managed at local levels throughout the NHS. These questions are best handled by writing about something you are familiar with, but try to avoid describing situations where you apportion blame to another person without justifying the causes. Risk management is not about pointing fingers; it is about identifying areas where risk exists and putting procedures in place to stop them from happening. Very few errors are down to one person alone, and are usually the result of multiple small errors at many levels. For example:

> On a recent ward round, after finishing a patient review, a junior colleague and I returned to the ward base to wash our hands. I noticed that the piece of paper in the patient's case notes, on which she had just documented our assessment, was labelled with the wrong patient sticker. As we investigated this matter, it became clear that the ward clerk had labelled several sheets of as-yet unused paper with the wrong patient stickers in error. My junior colleague and I had not checked the sticker at the top of the blank sheet. This was clearly a risk management issue and we discussed it with the ward clerk, the ward manager, our consultant and the patient. We filled in and submitted a critical incident form and discussed it at our regional clinical governance meeting. It transpired that the ward clerk had been under a significantly increased workload due to her colleague being off sick and had been under pressure from junior doctors to have the notes labelled and ready. The decision was taken that no pre-labelling should be performed on blank paper, and that in future it should be the responsibility of the persons documenting in the notes to check the correct details were there. An audit of selected case notes is now planned to ensure correct patient details are on all notes, in keeping with good record-keeping practice.

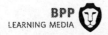

Commitment to specialty

A common question in recent years has centred on how you can give evidence of your commitment to your chosen specialty. This is obviously easier for the more senior trainees to demonstrate, but there are ways in which more junior doctors can display commitment:

- Establishing that you have chosen your elective and special study modules in subjects related to your chosen specialty gives evidence to the fact that you have given thought to your future career.
- Gaining specialty-specific exams and courses at an early stage also shows insight into the competition of the specialty.
- If you have relocated to pursue a particular job to further your career, this further demonstrates commitment as does shadowing and pursuit of specialty-specific experience outside of working hours.

For example, an applicant to a GP programme might put:

I have wanted to pursue a career in General Practice since Medical School and have chosen all of my projects and electives accordingly. I am highly motivated to continue my training in General Practice, having completed over twelve months in GP practices as part of my rotations, using each placement to further my career progression.

I have taken every opportunity to shadow the senior GPs at my practice during out-of-hours work, community clinics and home visits. I have performed several volunteer sessions at the community drop-in clinics and attended regional primary care meetings related to clinical governance. This has helped me gain considerable clinical and management experience.

I have completed a clinical audit relevant to General Practice, regarding the management of patients on methotrexate in primary care. I have published my work in peer-reviewed

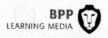

journals and attended national meetings. I have completed my MRCGP examination and relevant courses to equip me with skills required at ST3 level.

Other skills and achievements

The demonstration of a life outside of medicine is always a good thing. It proves that you have other interests and goals and ways to relax when work becomes stressful. As stated previously in this book, be honest when listing your hobbies and interests. There are always rumours circulating that particular hobbies score more points than others, ie fencing for hand-eye co-ordination or photography for spatial orientation. I am not certain that these are true and also for the one point it may gain on the form, it is not worth the worry and stress at having to learn fencing manoeuvres or shutter speeds. Keep it simple. For example:

I am a keen runner and have completed several ten-kilometre runs, most recently in October last year. I am currently training for my first half marathon.

I play the cello, enjoy horse riding and play the acoustic guitar. I enjoy cinema, chess and reading.

Relevant further information

Often there will be a section at the end of the form which asks you to include any information you feel is relevant to this application. This section is the equivalent of the Career intentions statement at the end of your CV. It is a good opportunity to slot in any parts of your CV which have not been covered by the earlier more structured sections, including your career intentions, your understanding of the demands of the specialty and any statements about yourself which you feel make you fit the person specification. Again, the right tone of confidence without arrogance must be struck here.

I wish to become an A&E trainee because of the clinical variety it provides, in terms of pathology, procedure and patient-group.

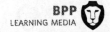

The combination of diagnostic thinking and hands-on emergency management appeals to me. I enjoy the teamwork involved in A&E and its interaction with other specialties.

I feel that I have a realistic view of a challenging and competitive specialty that can be extremely rewarding. I believe I fit the person specification for this training programme to a high degree, and have demonstrated aptitude, progression and suitability.

I am confident that I possess the personal and professional qualities vital to the progression of a good A&E trainee; I am hardworking, reliable and a good team player and intend to build on my current level of competencies to progress well through training.

Why this programme?

Finally, some forms will ask, 'Why this particular programme, in this particular region?' This requires a bit of background research into the specifics of the training programme applied for, or the region to which you are applying. A bit of knowledge about the regional teaching programme, the areas through which you will be expected to rotate and the specialist interests of the units involved (eg cancer research units, transplant centres, etc) is worthwhile. This information can usually be found on the deanery websites, but for more in-depth knowledge it may be worth contacting the people in the positions you are applying for. A word of warning here: do not leave this until the last minute, as many other people will have the same idea and you are likely to be met via the switchboard of the relevant hospital by a very grumpy-sounding doctor who is having a busy day on call and is fending off questions from nervous applicants who have left things until the last minute! Plan to do this early.

If you have friends or relatives in the area which make it more attractive for you then mention this; any connection with the region is something to talk about. However, do not wax lyrical about the 'lush beautiful green hills of Wales' being the reason

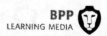

you are applying, as it sounds trite. If there are local attractions that are relevant to you and your interests then by all means say so. Make it justifiable but also honest! For example:

I am applying for this Specialty Training programme because I feel it would be an excellent place to train. The programme comes highly recommended by current trainees in your programme and senior colleagues at my unit. The specialist interests of the unit in terms of research work with gene therapy and the involvement in formation of national guidance interest me greatly. I feel that the rotation between the larger teaching hospitals and the district general units would provide a broad-based and varied level of experience at my stage of training.

My application to the Peninsula region is strengthened by the presence of my family in Penzance and my strong interest in surfing, in which I have competed at regional level. I know the area very well and feel I could be very happy living and training here.

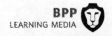

Chapter 7
ARCP/RITA

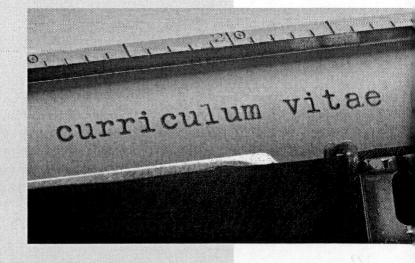

ARCP/RITA

Introduction

At every stage of your training there will always be an Annual Review of Clinical Performance (ARCP) or Record of In-Training Assessment (RITA) with designated consultants to assess your progress and performance throughout the year. This kind of review has had many names over the years, but the process has not changed essentially. The aim is to ensure that you have achieved the relevant clinical competencies for your stage of training, which are set at the beginning of the year via your Programme Director and Educational Supervisor. The review involves collating a large amount of information regarding your global progress during the year and will be based largely on evidence that you will be asked to provide in the form of a training portfolio. This training portfolio may be hard copy or online, and although current medical opinion favours the latter, it is always wise to keep a version of the former for your own records, keeping any paper documents you are given such as course certificates. This will always be a safeguard in the event of any technical failures.

The portfolio is not a new concept and has long been used in many professions as a method of recording evidence of your personal and professional skills, knowledge and competencies. As mentioned in the Introduction, with the recent changes evident in medical training it has never been more important to keep a well-presented and comprehensive record of the skills, qualities and competencies necessary to present at these reviews. The review will often consist of a panel of consultants from several hospitals throughout the region, some or all of whom you may not be acquainted with. Therefore, the information in the portfolio you present is likely to be the only information that these assessors will have on which to base their decision regarding your progression to the next level, and its importance is not to be underestimated.

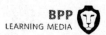

Once again, the importance of adequate preparation cannot be overemphasised. You may be the best trainee in the region, but appearing at your Annual Review with a few sheets of paper and a wry grin is not going to work; you will embarrass yourself and those who have helped you in your career. These people are putting their signatures next to a document that is going to allow you to advance your career, and they will require adequate reassurance that their faith in doing this is justified.

Your portfolio will also be used when you meet your Educational Supervisor at the beginning of a job, particularly to look back at your previous training jobs and to see where areas that need development exist. This is essential, as setting you an educational or training goal which you have already achieved is a waste of everyone's time, and with the reduction of doctors' working hours in recent years, particularly since 2009, every training opportunity is essential to ensure that you achieve the desired goals and experience in a relatively short period. Helping your Educational Supervisor by presenting him or her with a clear and logical portfolio of what you have done before this job is going to show that you are organised, resourceful and keen. He or she is also likely to be grateful to you for making their job a little easier and at the risk of sounding calculating, this is always good when you are asking for a reference.

Finally, job interviews are also likely to require you to bring your portfolio with you for review. When registering for the interview, the administration team will usually ask you to hand them your portfolio and give it to the interview panel for review before you enter the interview room, to let the panel target their questions effectively. As interviews always run on a very tight schedule, there is often only five minutes or so for the panel to look at your portfolio, therefore the production of a neat and logical portfolio that clearly outlines your skills and experience can only gain you points with the panel and increase your chances of securing the position. At several interviews I have attended, I have seen a smart and confident candidate arrive, and when asked for their portfolio, produce a scruffy looking

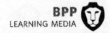

sheaf of paper in a plastic wallet. This had the joint effect of making me feel sorry for them but also making me think my chances of interview success had just improved. One interview I attended asked me to prepare a five-minute presentation on 'The Importance of a Surgical Portfolio'. This question could easily have applied to any specialty and can only highlight the relevance of the portfolio in modern interviews.

Preparation

There is no point in knowing how to construct an excellent portfolio if when the time comes to present your evidence, you find you do not have enough of it. Strictly speaking you should be collating evidence in the forms of competency-based assessments, logbook procedures and reflective practice, for example, all through the year. In reality, many of us are too busy to do this on a monthly basis. Therefore it is advisable to put reminders in your paper or electronic organiser at the start of the year, at say three-monthly intervals to remind you to review your portfolio and see if there are areas in which you are slipping. Again, this seems like a lot of hard work and perhaps even overkill, but the stress of trying to gather a year's worth of training evidence the week before a review or interview is horrible, and often it is obvious that you have not kept things up-to-date (ie dates on assessments and logbooks are all suspiciously similar).

Key preparation points

- Try to keep on top of all your workplace-based competency assessments (DOPS/mini-CEX/CBD/PBA). These will be discussed in detail later in the chapter. If you are going to assess a potentially interesting patient, try to get your senior to come and watch you to make it a mini-CEX. If you are about to perform a procedure with a senior colleague, then ask them in advance if they can treat this as a DOPS/PBA and meet with you afterwards to fill in the assessment form. Ring your consultant's secretary and ask if you can book a half-hour slot for a CBD (after asking them if this is ok, of course), meaning there is a specific time set aside for you to do this.

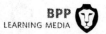

- Keep a record of the teaching sessions you attend over the year and the subjects and areas involved along with the dates you attended. Trying to get this information seven months down the line is near impossible and takes a lot of time.
- Keep a record of any teaching you deliver and try to get some form of feedback in terms of a feedback form or questionnaire, or even just post-it notes with good points and suggestions for improvement. This will not only provide evidence of the teaching delivered, but show that you are critical in your practice and taking steps to assess and review your teaching performance at every stage.

Key portfolio construction points

- Use a large dark-coloured ring binder. This will ensure it is conservative enough not to offend anyone. This may sound pedantic, but think of it in terms of representing you as a trainee. Even if you feel that the bright shiny pink plastic folder is pretty and reflects your personality, as a trainee serious about progression perhaps matt burgundy suede would be more appropriate. In addition, dark colours hide scuffs and marks better which will mean it needs replacing less often.
- Have at least eight section dividers and lots of plastic wallets.
- Create a Contents page to be placed in a plastic wallet and kept at the front of your portfolio. This will make it easier for the reviewer to find the evidence they are looking for quickly, maximising the time available for them to do your portfolio justice.
- Place two up-to-date copies of your CV after the Contents page. This will ensure that if the reviewer or interviewer wishes to peruse it, they can do so and take a copy to keep with your information, leaving one behind. If you are at an interview where they ask you not to include a CV in your portfolio, you can always remove it.
- Keep photocopies of your essential documents like your degree certificate, your GMC certificate and your passport in a plastic wallet at the back of your portfolio. You will often be informed as to which document copies to bring for review or interview, but being prepared will avoid the occasional long queues at the photocopier with other trainees/candidates.

Constructing the portfolio

The General Medical Council outlines the pillars of Good Medical Practice, to which all doctors at all stages of training should

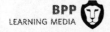

adhere, in the document entitled *Good Medical Practice* (2006) on the GMC website. This is worth a read, as it is the basis from which all the standards by which doctors should be measured have been described. The GMC outline the definition of a good doctor as follows:

> *Good doctors make the care of their patients their first concern: they are competent, keep their knowledge and skills up to date, establish and maintain good relationships with patients and colleagues, are honest and trustworthy, and act with integrity.*

This statement summarises the pillars of Good Medical Practice. In order to prove to any reviewer or interviewer that you are a good doctor in whichever specialty you have chosen, you must be able to prove that you fulfil the criteria outlined in this document. It makes sense, therefore, to divide the contents of your portfolio into the seven pillars of Good Medical Practice, which are listed below:

1. Good clinical care
2. Maintaining good medical practice
3. Teaching and training, appraising and assessing
4. Relationships with patients
5. Working with colleagues
6. Probity
7. Health

By displaying your portfolio in this manner you are showing that not only do you have evidence in each pillar of Good Medical Practice that you are a good doctor, but also that you have considered the standards of the GMC by which you are being continually measured and have organised your portfolio in a logical manner. There may be some sections where you have very little evidence to add, simply because very little evidence is required, but it shows that you are thinking about these pillars in every area of your practice.

 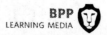

Looking at each of the Good Medical Practice pillars individually, we can determine what evidence is suitable for each pillar. A brief outline of the principles of each pillar is included. If you are organising your portfolio this way it would be prudent to know some of the principles well enough to answer any questions at review or interview, and reading the full details of the pillars on the General Medical Council's website is advised.

Good clinical care

Providing good clinical care is an extremely broad topic encompassing many of the duties of a doctor. In providing good clinical care, you must be able to:

- Adequately assess the patient, arrange investigations, treatment or further advice or referral
- Recognise your limitations, consulting senior colleagues if necessary
- Provide optimum care based on the best possible evidence
- Alleviate pain and discomfort
- Respect the patient's right to a second opinion
- Keep legible, comprehensive and accurate records
- Be readily available when on duty
- Encourage patients to be aware of and maintain/improve their health status
- Avoid treating those close to you
- Raise concerns immediately if patient safety is compromised in any way
- Do not let your own personal/political/religious/moral beliefs deny a patient care – if you cannot provide the patient with the required care then you must refer the patient to a colleague
- Do not deny a patient treatment if their medical condition may put you at risk – try to minimise risk or make other arrangements
- Offer assistance in cases of emergency

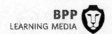

Using these broad statements as a guide, you can now select the parts of your portfolio which are applicable to this particular pillar. It is obvious that the majority of the evidence here will relate to your workplace competency-based assessments, which are listed below with brief explanations. These assessments are obviously all different when relating to different specialties – an assessment relevant to an Obstetrics and Gynaecology trainee would obviously need adjustment for a Psychiatry trainee. For details, see the individual Royal College websites and the Postgraduate Medical Education and Training Board (PMETB) website.

Mini-Clinical Evaluation Exercise (Mini-CEX)

The mini-CEX broadly assesses a trainee in the elements of history-taking, physical examination, communication skills, clinical judgment, professionalism and efficiency. The trainee will be scored in each of these domains and then an overall mark given. Over a year, the guidance estimates the minimum number of mini-CEXs a trainee should have is six (two for each four-month placement, three for each six-month placement and six for a year's placement), but in reality more are desirable.

Direct Observation of Procedural Skills (DOPS)

DOPS assesses a trainee in terms of their technical, professional and/or operative skills in a variety of procedures, which depending on the relevant specialty can be used to assess a range of diagnostic, interventional or operational procedures. There are specific DOPS that are assigned for each level of training in each specialty, but there is some scope for flexibility as you can add the name of the procedure performed yourself. As with mini-CEX there are marks assigned to particular parts of the procedure including gaining informed consent, safe use of sharps and clear post-procedural instructions. Then there is an overall mark for the ability to complete the procedure. Over a year, similar to the mini-CEX, six DOPS should be the minimum performed; however, as DOPS are relatively quick and easy to perform you should try to get as many as possible.

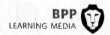

Case Based Discussion (CBD)

The case based discussion should be performed with a consultant, reviewing over a set of case notes a particular case in which you have been involved. The aim of this is to assess the trainee's ability to prioritise and make clinical judgments and decisions using the application of their knowledge to a situation. It focuses on scoring the domains of record-keeping, assessment, investigation, treatment, follow-up, professionalism and clinical judgment. Again, there is an overall mark given. The number of CBDs required over a year is less, with a minimum of three recommended (one for each four-month placement, one or two for each six-month placement).

Procedure Based Assessment (PBA)

These are more specific versions of DOPS for specific procedures/operations and usually only relevant for those trainees at registrar level or above, as completion of a PBA indicates a level of competence to perform that procedure independently. It goes in far more detail into each of the domains of consent, pre-operative/procedural planning and preparation, operative/procedural technique and post-operative/procedural management, with an overall score applied, indicating a level of competence. Guidance of the number of PBAs that should be performed varies depending on the level of the trainee, but discussion with your educational supervisor at the beginning of a placement should help to clarify what is expected of you. What is important to remember is that you do not have to be competent in all areas of the operation or procedure to complete a section of the PBA. For example, in a common general surgical operation such as appendicectomy, you may be able to demonstrate definite competence in the opening of the abdomen or insertion of laparoscopic ports, and therefore have your supervisor complete part of the PBA form to evidence this, whilst you continue to work on your experience with the rest of the procedure.

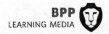

Special note

Currently, things differ between specialties as to how the results of these workplace-based assessments are seen. Many specialties have online training logs where you can upload these assessments for viewing and consolidation. However, some deaneries still rely on hard copies to be presented at review. In either case, you are unlikely to have access to your online training record at interview. The point of this is that these assessments viewed singularly are of very little benefit; what the panel of any review or interview wants to see are trends and evidence of progression. In other words, they want to see that you have improved in your scores in all of these assessments over the year.

The best way to do this (although it requires a little work, preparation and patience) is to make a graph of your progress. For example, for a particular DOPS procedure relevant to your specialty, say excision of skin lesion or arterial line insertion, you may have six DOPS on this procedure over a twelve-month period. Take the overall scores for the DOPS on each assessment and make a bar chart in chronological date order (Microsoft Excel can easily help you do this) to show that you have maintained or improved your score standards over this period of time. This is a simple and effective way of clearly displaying to the panel that you have progressed during your year's training and have the evidence to prove it. This method can be similarly applied for PBAs for more advanced surgeons, mini-CEX (eg respiratory examination) for medical trainees, and so on. Yes, it is a lot of effort, but it shows initiative and a desire to progress, admirable qualities in trainees for any specialty.

Logbook

Include a consolidated version of your entire logbook in a plastic wallet and then one that has a filter applied for the past year, or the time period that this assessment is reviewing. This will let the reviewers/interviewers see your global experience, but also and more importantly, what you have achieved during the past year during the relevant time period.

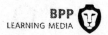

Maintaining good medical practice

Maintaining 'good medical practice' refers to a doctor's responsibility to keep up to date in terms of the knowledge and skill-base essential to perform their work. This is explained more fully in the GMC website document *Continuing Professional Development (CPD)*. CPD as a concept links closely with maintenance of good medical practice, encompassing lifelong learning and a commitment to keeping up to date throughout your working life. To maintain good medical practice a doctor should:

- Keep abreast of relevant clinical guidelines and developments that affect your work
- Complete regular educational activities to maintain and improve your knowledge and competence
- Be aware of and comply with laws and codes of practice relevant to your work
- Keep a portfolio
- Reflect on your practice
- Involve yourself in clinical audit, quality assurance and improvement
- Promote patient safety, in particular with regard to adverse event recognition and inquiries

Documents to include in this section are as follows.

GMC certificate/Degree certificate/Medical Indemnity certificate

These essential certificates need to be kept in your portfolio, particularly for interview scenarios. Include here any higher degree certificates also, as these are evidence of your efforts to maintain and improve your medical practice.

Educational contracts

Most training jobs require you to complete an educational contract with your assigned educational supervisor, either in

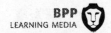

hard copy or online. This outlines an agreement between you that you will fulfil the requirements of a trainee and in turn will be provided with the opportunities for training. Include a copy of your current educational contract (print one out if it has been completed online). This is evidence that you have made the effort to complete this essential document and have considered your training needs and taken responsibility for your training.

Foundation Achievement of Competency Document (FACD) or equivalent

For trainees who have completed a Foundation programme, this is easy to produce, as you will have been issued with a FACD at the end of your programme. However, if you graduated before this system was introduced, you have to provide evidence of your equivalent competence in whatever programme you completed. For example, this might be evidence that you completed an educationally approved house-officer job in the UK, your completed House Officer Training Log or a statement from your deanery or Educational Supervisor in that post attesting to your Foundation competencies.

RITA/ARCP certificates

Provide all previous annual assessment certificates of whatever form is applicable to your stage of training. List these, as with everything, in reverse chronological order, so that the reviewers can quickly see that you passed last year's assessment.

Learning agreements

As with the educational contract, modern trainees must now fill out a specific learning agreement with their assigned educational supervisor within the first few weeks of the post to set educational objectives for them to complete during their current post. These will obviously be different depending on how long you will be in the post and your current level of training and previous experience. As mentioned, bringing your portfolio to such meetings is advantageous. Every specialty will have different

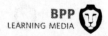

kinds of well-defined objectives set out by the specialty Royal College and these meetings involve the selection of relevant objectives and plans as to how you will fulfil them. File paper copies of your learning objectives over the past year, so that you can demonstrate how you have achieved these if asked. Again, file in reverse chronological order.

Personal Development Plan (PDP)

The construction of your learning objectives is based on your PDP. It is different to a learning agreement – a PDP is a self-assessment of your own training needs whilst your learning agreement is the construction, with your educational supervisor, of specific objectives that you will achieve over a period of time. If your training is working then you will be continuously achieving your learning objectives, which alters your PDP over the year and specifically after each placement is completed. There may be a specific PDP available on your Royal College's website, but if not there is a version on the MMC website (www.mmc. nhs.uk) which you can use as a template. These PDPs centre around three questions:

- What specific developmental needs do I have?
- How will these objectives be addressed?
- How will I show I have achieved my objectives?

Filling in and filing a PDP not only shows that you have done one, but also that you are keeping it in your portfolio as a reminder of your developmental needs and the ways in which you are attempting to attain them. To give a very simple example, a GP trainee may identify their developmental need to progress with specialty examinations. This objective will be addressed by registering for and revising for the exam and making use of appropriate resources such as departmental and regional teaching sessions, exam revision courses and study groups. They will show that they have achieved their objective by passing the examination and producing the certificate in their portfolio. Another example might be a Specialty Registrar in Paediatrics,

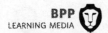

who identifies a specific training need to gain competence in the procedure of lumbar puncture. The objective will be addressed by watching senior colleagues perform the procedure, revising their knowledge of the relevant anatomy and complications, attending A&E on-call and asking senior colleagues to supervise them in their attempts to perform the procedure when they feel confident enough. The trainee will show that they have achieved their objective by the production of DOPS and PBA forms in Paediatric Lumbar Puncture and the record of such procedures completed in their logbook.

Reflective practice

Reflective practice is very popular at present, and its inclusion in a portfolio shows that you are aware of the current guidance in line with the GMC and MMC regarding the best way to learn. I once tried to explain to a visiting Belgian colleague the fundamentals of reflective practice and he asked 'So you actually *highlight* your failings to your assessors? You're mad!' It might appear that this is the case, but reflective practice is about looking at an area of your practice in the form of a particular situation that was relevant educationally, legally, ethically or personally. The aim is to identify what made the experience relevant, how it affected you, the patient and the team, identifying what you learned from the situation and if there was anything that you would do differently if confronted with a similar situation in the future. Again, your specialty may provide specific forms for this on their Royal College website, but there is a downloadable version of a generic reflective practice form on the MMC website. Reflective practice is not only good medical practice, it is evidence that you have the ability to look at a situation and appraise it critically, looking at how it has affected those involved and how it will shape your future practice. The MMC guidance suggests you should take time every day to do this, reflecting on your day's events. However, the inclusion of three or four reflective practice forms for each placement is probably sufficient and as always should be filed in reverse chronological order and be completely anonymous, so as to protect confidentiality of patients

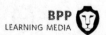

and staff involved. For example, a Psychiatry or GP trainee may reflect upon a home visit to a patient with schizophrenia where it became apparent that the patient had deteriorated significantly and required admission via the process of Section 4 of the Mental Health Act for acute assessment. They could perhaps describe any uncomfortable moments with the patient or their relatives and how this made them feel. They could describe the effect on the patient, and how the Mental Health team handling the situation felt it had gone. Finally they could record what they learnt from the situation in terms of how to proceed with a Community Section order and any areas where they would proceed differently in the future. However, there do not need to be areas which you would perform differently, it just needs to be an event that was significant to you or the patient and something you can reflect upon and learn.

Examination results

Part of maintaining good medical practice is the continuation of your learning, which must include the attainment of Royal College examinations. Include your certificate or your official results papers from the college here, even if you have only passed part of the examination so far. It is evidence that you are progressing and achieving the qualifications needed for advancement in your field.

Publications and presentations

Publishing articles and presenting research or audit is strong evidence of continuing your medical education and contributing to the knowledge of the medical community. Include copies of all your publications (most recent first) and either the listing or summary of your presentation at the relevant scientific meeting or if this is not available a paper copy of the slides of your talk, (made more compact if needed by having six slides to a piece of A4 paper). Reviewers and interviewers alike will want to see these to prove that you have indeed published and/or presented your work.

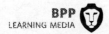

Audits

Evidence of participation in clinical audit is mandatory from the level of Foundation training onwards and also forms part of Clinical Governance, so ensure that you have something to display in this section. Foundation trainees must perform at least one audit during their training and specialty trainees should really have evidence of their involvement in one audit a year. Include copies of the presentation or write-up of your most recent audits. If these have changed practice at your unit, try to include evidence of this. For example, if your audit resulted in the inclusion of a checklist for a procedure or departmental handbook/guideline then file a copy with the audit.

Course/meeting certificates

Attendance at courses, training days and scientific meetings is all evidence of maintaining good medical practice and Continuing Professional Development. File the completion certificates from all relevant courses and meetings in reverse chronological order. In order to save space and to avoid making your portfolio too bulky you can use one plastic wallet to display two certificates, one on either side.

Teaching

Evidence of attendance at a regional or departmental teaching programme is desirable, and can be helped by providing a summary of the topics covered and the dates the teaching was delivered. File a typed copy of the summary of teaching you have attended in the last year here; it looks professional and shows you are keeping up-to-date with your learning by identifying what you have already covered in some depth. It is also useful to justify any areas of your objectives that you have not yet managed to get around to. For example, if as a Plastic Surgery trainee, you could be asked at your ARCP why you have 'Improve knowledge of Cleft Palate Conditions and Sequelae' as one of your learning objectives, yet have no workplace-based assessments or logbook evidence of operations on this topic. There

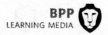

may be perfectly reasonable explanations for this, eg you work in an adult hospital and have not yet rotated to paediatric cover. However it is far better to be able to show you have attended a teaching session on this subject, gone home and reflected, and now plan to shadow a senior colleague at the Children's Hospital to rectify this.

Self-directed teaching

There are various methods of displaying evidence of your own efforts to enhance your knowledge. One of the most popular are e-learning modules via web-based sites such as doctors.net, where you can enter your specialty and training level and see relevant modules in subjects that may not be covered regularly in your own teaching programme (eg major incident plan scenarios, current thromboprophylaxis guidelines). Completion of these educational activities awards the doctor 'CPD hours' in recognition of the time spent to complete them and provides a printable certificate on completion. Be aware however, the certificates show the date they were completed and if you have seven of these all completed the week before your review/interview, it will not look as impressive as if they are spread throughout the year.

Teaching and training, appraising and assessing

The GMC highlights that the teaching and training of junior colleagues and students is important for the maintenance of high standards in both present and future care and states that doctors should be willing to give their support in these educational activities. To provide good quality teaching and training you should:

- Develop necessary skills and attitudes for a teacher
- Provide adequate supervision for all staff for whom you are responsible
- Be honest and impartial when assessing or appraising colleagues in order to maintain the highest levels of patient safety

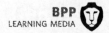

- Be honest and accurate when providing a report regarding, or a reference for, a colleague

Teaching experience

If you have any evidence of formal teaching delivered previously then include it here, although experience prior to Medical School, whilst probably still relevant for CVs and application forms is probably a little out-of-date for your portfolio. The more recent the teaching, the more relevant it is. File a typed summary of teaching sessions you have delivered and include copies of any handouts you have made for teaching sessions and feedback forms on your performance.

Relationships with patients

Maintaining good, ethical and honest relationships with your patients is a non-negotiable part of GMC dogma. A doctor's first responsibility is to make the care of their patients their first concern. Such a relationship will allow you to work optimally with your patients together to address any health issues they may have. In maintaining good relationships with patients you must:

- Be honest, considerate and polite, treat patients as individuals and with dignity
- Encourage patients to be involved with their health and decisions that affect their care
- Listen to patients' views, concerns and preferences and respect their rights to privacy and confidentiality
- Share with patients information about their condition and treatment, respond to their questions and keep them informed
- Make arrangements to meet patients' language and communication needs
- Protect the health and well-being of children, young people and vulnerable groups, treat them with respect and listen to their views, answer their questions and provide information they can understand

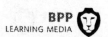

- Be considerate and supportive to patients' partners, carers and relatives, providing information whilst respecting patients' confidentiality
- Be honest and open if things have gone wrong or a complaint has been made
- Do not abuse your professional position to pursue a sexual or improper relationship with a patient or patient's carer/relative/partner
- Do not express your own personal, moral, political or religious beliefs to a patient in a way to exploit them or cause them distress
- Ensure you have adequate professional indemnity and are identifiable to your patients via your registered name and GMC number
- Obtain valid and informed consent before undertaking any examination, investigation, research or procedure
- If you feel the need to end a professional relationship with a patient, ensure that your decision is fair and not based on a patient's complaint, and arrange for the prompt continuation of that patient's care by another practitioner

It is difficult to provide evidence that you form good relationships with your patients. Lack of complaints is hardly an area you can prove, and doesn't really prove anything anyway, as they might feel intimidated by you! You can however, indicate that you follow the guidance regarding dealing with patients, particularly with the inclusion of reflective practice. Below are some pieces of evidence that you can include here, but try to get a feeling of how well you have communicated with your patient by their responses to you and the feedback that they give the nurses, which is often the healthcare group with whom the patients are most honest.

'Thank you' cards

It is always nice to receive a thank you card from a patient. Whilst by no means expected, it makes you feel that your hard work has been recognised and your relationship with your patient

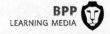

successful and always lifts your day. These cards are also good evidence of your ability to provide good care and form the kind of professional relationship with a patient where they want to thank you for it. Include your cards here, with the names blanked out with black pen, so as to maintain the confidentiality of the thoughtful patient who wrote it.

Reflective practice

Reflective practice is again relevant here. If you have been especially pleased with the communication between yourself and a patient, or there has been a particularly trying encounter which you tried to resolve, record it here. Evidence that you are thinking about assessing and improving your patient relationships is almost as important as the type of relationship you have with them. For example, there may have been a recent time where you broke some bad news, or explained a treatment to a patient for the first time. It does not have to be groundbreaking stuff, just relevant to you personally and something you can reflect upon.

Relationships with colleagues

Maintaining good working relationships with your colleagues is essential for Good Medical Practice, as teamwork and communication between colleagues is vital for delivering good patient care and maintaining a healthy working life. You must:

- Respect the contributions and skills of your colleagues
- Communicate with them effectively and treat them with respect
- Ensure your role and responsibilities in the team are defined
- Take part in regular reviews and audit of the team's performance
- Support colleagues who have problems
- Protect patients from any threat posed by a colleague's conduct or performance, including taking steps to protect

patients if a colleague is not fit to practise, following local guidance or regulatory bodies

- Do not bully or discriminate against your colleagues
- Arrange suitable cover for when you are going to be off duty
- Take up any post formally accepted and work required notice before leaving a department
- When referring a patient, provide relevant details including their current condition and medical history
- Keep the patient's General Practitioner informed regarding the specifics of their patient's condition including investigations and treatment
- If delegating or referring care, ensure the person to whom you are delegating or referring is qualified and experienced enough to care for the patient

Self Mini-PAT/Mini-PAT

Providing evidence of your working relationship with colleagues used to rely solely on the reference from your consultant. However, in the creation of workplace-based assessments, it was considered that a more well-rounded and multi-disciplinary style feedback would be more appropriate. This led to the development of the Multi-Source Feedback Tool; also known as a 360-degree assessment or a Mini-Peer Assessment Tool (Mini-PAT). This tool requires ten trainee-nominated assessors, from a range of doctor training levels and multi-disciplinary healthcare professional disciplines, to score the doctor in all pillars of Good Medical Practice against the standards expected for a doctor at their level of training. The Self Mini-PAT is the same assessment form, but requires doctors to rate themselves. The online submission of these forms, via the relevant specialty body, produces a graph where the trainee can see where they have rated themselves and the scores their assessors have given them. Trainees must undertake one mini-PAT during their Foundation years and at least two during their Specialty Training. File your completed mini-PAT reports here as evidence that you have completed them and also to (hopefully) display to your reviewers/interviewers

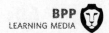

that members of the multi-disciplinary team in which you work have rated you favourably.

'Goodbye'/'Good luck' cards

As with the patient thank you cards, 'goodbye and good luck' cards from members of your previous teams evidence the fact that you have enjoyed a good working relationship with them.

Probity

Probity encompasses the qualities of honesty and integrity and used in terms of Good Medical Practice relates to a trustworthy doctor. This is an important part of Good Medical Practice and any breach in probity is taken very seriously by the GMC. To ensure you are acting with probity you must:

- Act with conduct that justifies the patient and public trust in you
- Inform the GMC about any cautions, investigations or charges against you by the police or other professional body
- Publish factual and original work
- Be honest and open when writing reports or documents
- Be honest regarding your qualifications, experience and positions
- Co-operate fully and confidentially with any inquiry or complaints
- Assist the Coroner or Procurator Fiscal in any inquest or inquiry
- Act with integrity when performing research, protecting patients' interests first, following national research governance and guidance
- Be honest and open regarding any financial arrangements with patients
- Be honest in financial and commercial dealings with employers, insurers, organisations and individuals

Statement of probity

Most training programmes will ask you as a trainee to fill in a statement of probity prior to commencing each training placement, either in hard-copy or online, confirming that you accept the professional obligations of the training programme and that you have no undisclosed convictions or disciplinary action/investigation against you. This should be kept up-to-date, signed and filed here as a record of your agreement with this statement.

Criminal Records Bureau (CRB) disclosure

Include a copy of your most recent CRB disclosure to allow reviewers and future employers to see that you take the issue of probity seriously and have this vital document, which is necessary to work independently in the NHS.

Reflective practice

Again, if there have been any situations relating to probity that you have been involved in, recording a statement of reflective practice here shows that you consider this important element of Good Medical Practice in your day-to-day working life. An example of this world be any instances when performing research where you have questioned the ethics of proceeding with a study and the measures you have taken to ensure you are proceeding secure in the knowledge that your probity is unaffected.

Health

Maintaining your own health as a doctor is essential to ensure that you are fit to work. There are certain standards of health that are requisite for a doctor and keeping yourself healthy is your responsibility. You must:

- Register with a General Practitioner outside of your family to ensure you have objective medical care
- Protect your patients and colleagues by ensuring you are

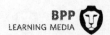

immunised against serious communicable diseases for which vaccines are available

- Consult a colleague or Occupational Health if you think you have a serious condition that could be transmitted to patients or where your judgement or performance may be impaired by it or its treatment

Health declaration

As with the probity statement, you are likely to be required to complete a health declaration at the start of your training placement, requiring you to confirm that you are not under any medical supervision or restriction as the result of an illness or condition. Make sure you have an up-to-date copy signed and filed to show your compliance with this and your recognition of its importance.

Health passport

All trainees should keep copies of their health record, usually called a health passport, as it travels with you from hospital to hospital to prove that you are sufficiently immunised and do not have any undisclosed communicable diseases. If you do not have a copy of these records you can request a copy from your hospital's Occupational Health department. This essential health information should be filed here.

Additional Continuing Professional Development (CPD) evidence

There are always pieces of evidence that do not fit clearly into any one particular category. If relevant these should always be included as they are still evidence of Continuing Professional Development. These could include evidence of foreign language study, outstanding achievements in sports or other interests outside of medicine, evidence of extra experience in your chosen specialty or particular specialty commitment (for example, any Higher Degree modules in which you performed particularly well, Royal College Awards or Prizes, Fellowship reports,

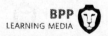

etc). File these here in reverse chronological order so that the individuals reviewing your portfolio can see the most recent and relevant quickly.

Checklist summary

Good clinical care
- ☑ Mini-CEX (with summary chart if possible)
- ☑ DOPS (with summary chart if possible)
- ☑ CBD
- ☑ PBA (with summary chart if possible)
- ☑ Logbook

Maintaining good medical practice
- ☑ GMC/Degree/Medical Indemnity certificates
- ☑ Educational contracts
- ☑ Foundation Achievement or equivalent
- ☑ RITA/ARCP certificates
- ☑ Learning agreements
- ☑ Personal Development Plan
- ☑ Reflective practice (for each placement)
- ☑ Examination results
- ☑ Publications and presentations
- ☑ Audits
- ☑ Course meeting certificates
- ☑ Teaching attendance summary
- ☑ Self-directed teaching

Teaching and training, appraising and assessing
- ☑ Summary of teaching delivered with feedback if possible
- ☑ Formal teaching delivered

Relationships with patients
- ☑ Patient informal feedback (thank you cards)
- ☑ Reflective practice

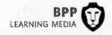

Relationships with colleagues
- ☑ Self mini-PAT
- ☑ Multi-Source Feedback/360 degree assessments
- ☑ Goodbye/good luck cards

Probity
- ☑ Statement of probity
- ☑ CRB disclosure
- ☑ Reflective practice

Health
- ☑ Health declaration
- ☑ Health passport

Additional CPD evidence
- ☑ Extra-curricular achievements
- ☑ Evidence of specialty experience/commitment

By organising your portfolio in this manner you will be able to provide clearly and quickly the evidence needed to answer common questions asked at review/interview, 'How can you prove you are a good doctor?' and 'How can you demonstrate progression over this time period?' You have followed clear GMC guidance to reflect all areas of Good Medical Practice in your portfolio.

We all have evidence that we are good at what we do. To maximise our potential we need to display this evidence in a manner that can be seen quickly and clearly in a time-pressured situation.

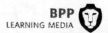

Chapter 8
Revalidation

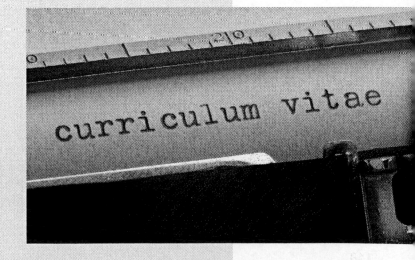

Revalidation

Introduction

Revalidation is a process that has been under development for some time now, whereby doctors will have to regularly display evidence to the GMC that they are competent, fit to practice and up to date. The concept of revalidation was introduced after the publication of several key documents listed below, which I recommend you read (www.dh.gov.uk/health/category/publications/reports-Publications):

- Good Doctors, Safer Patients: Proposals to strengthen the system to assure and improve the performance of doctors and to protect the safety of patients (Chief Medical Officer, 2006)
- Implementing the White Paper: Trust, Assurance and Safety: enhancing confidence in healthcare professional regulators (Department of Health, 2007)
- Medical revalidation – principles and next steps (Chief Medical Officer, 2008)

These publications centred on the improvement of patient safety by fortifying the regulation of doctors and reinforcing Continuing Professional Development, Multi-Source Feedback and specialty-specific standards. Basically, there must be a system by which the GMC can be satisfied on a regular basis that all doctors are upholding the pillars of Good Medical Practice and meeting clinical standards set by their specialty.

The process of revalidation is evolving even now; I cannot stress this strongly enough. The principles are outlined, but specifics are not yet finalised and the information that follows is correct at the time of writing. Details regarding revalidation may change, as the process is subject to pilots in order to ensure that the system works. Pilots of the specific processes required for revalidation have already been undertaken and pilots of the entire process having started this year (2011) with plans to

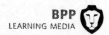

fully launch revalidation set for late 2012. Refer to the GMC website and the Revalidation Support Team website for updates at regular intervals.

The overall process of revalidation is to be achieved by two separate subsidiary processes: relicensing and recertification.

Relicensing

All doctors practising in the United Kingdom in the public or private sector will need a licence to practise, to be renewed every five years. The principle of relicensing is to ensure that all doctors are upholding the pillars of Good Medical Practice in their work, which will need to be demonstrated to the GMC. This will consist of three core elements:

- Annual appraisal (based on your portfolio)
- Multi-source feedback from patients and colleagues
- Confirmation from your healthcare organisation's Responsible Officer that there are no concerns

Recertification

All doctors on the General Practice or Specialist registers will need to recertify, again every five years, to demonstrate to the GMC and their Royal College that they are maintaining their specialty-specific standards. This is significant, as obviously there will be different standards for each specialty and different ways of measuring them. These standards, their measurement processes and the amount of evidence required will be individually decided by the relevant Royal Colleges for each specialty. The details of the formation of these standards have not yet been decided and a collaboration between the medical Royal Colleges and the GMC, known as The Academy of Medical Royal Colleges, has been formed to aid this process.

These two processes are not independent of one another and will form a single process by which a doctor can revalidate.

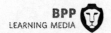

The evidence for both processes will be taken from the annual appraisals that every doctor must attend, with collation of this evidence after five years. This will result in the submission of evidence to a Responsible Officer in the healthcare organisation. The specifics regarding who this will be have not been decided finally, and may vary between England, Scotland, Wales and Northern Ireland, but the Responsible Officer will be a Licensed Medical Practitioner, probably be a senior member of medical staff such as the Medical Director. This Responsible Officer will then, based on the evidence presented for the five years, make a recommendation to the GMC as to whether a doctor should be relicensed, and also recertified if on the General Practice/Specialist register.

Revalidation and the training portfolio

The significance of revalidation is clear to all doctors. What is also clear is that the annual appraisals (see Chapter 7) will be the most important segment of evidence that you can provide to ensure that you are relicensed and recertified, and therefore maintaining a high-standard portfolio at these appraisals, which accurately reflects your high standards of work and practice, is more essential than ever. What is also clear is that doctors will need to display evidence and competence spread over the five years between revalidation dates – it will not be acceptable to have a 'fallow' year and then make up for it the year after.

The construction of your portfolio for the annual appraisals should still follow the guidance set out in Chapter 7, however, the GMC guidance has redesigned the display of evidence of Good Medical Practice at these five-yearly assessments into four domains:

1. Domain 1: Knowledge, skills and performance
2. Domain 2: Safety and quality
3. Domain 3: Communication, partnership and teamwork
4. Domain 4: Maintaining trust

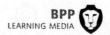

It is clear to see that these domains still encompass all of the evidence of Good Medical Practice, and where they relate to the original seven pillars, but have been redesigned into four broader areas combining elements of different pillars, termed a framework. There have also been some newer introductions, for example specific sections which apply to those doctors with a managerial or research role. The role of Multi-Source Feedback has also been examined, as aside from complaints there are no structured formal procedures by which patients can provide feedback on the care they receive from doctors. Draft questionnaires have been designed by the Peninsula Deanery for both colleagues and patients to fill in about a doctor's performance (these are available to view on the GMC website, www.gmc-uk.org/doctors/revalidation/9575.asp) and whilst these are still being piloted it is clear that formal patient and colleague feedback will form a significant part of the process of revalidation. Another part of Good Medical Practice that will receive increased emphasis in revalidation is reflective practice. This will extend to most parts of Continuing Professional Development. For example if you attend a training course or an educational activity, it will no longer be enough to simply attend. You will be required to reflect upon how it has altered, or will alter, your practice.

Again, as in Chapter 7: ARCP/RITA, the newer framework *Good Medical Practice* guidance is summarised below but all of this information is available in more detail on the GMC website under the heading of 'Revalidation'. It is essential to remember that this is an evolving process and that things may change before the introduction of revalidation, and keeping up-to-date with any possible changes is vital. With these domains in mind, it may be prudent to re-organise your portfolio in the following way for the revalidation purpose:

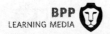

Domain 1: Knowledge, skills and performance

Maintain professional performance:

- Maintain up-to-date knowledge and skills; continue regular educational activities, audit and CPD; maintain knowledge of relevant laws and regulations

Apply knowledge and experience to practice:

- Undertake adequate assessment, advice, investigations and treatments for patients, prescribe appropriately and safely and provide optimum care based on the best possible evidence. Support patients in caring for themselves and, if appropriate, discuss cases with or refer patients to colleagues
- Recognise and work within limitations, follow national research governance guidelines, work effectively as a manager and teacher

Keep clear, accurate and legible records:

- Record legible, accurate and clear records of clinical findings, decision and delivered information at the same time or soon after the event.

This domain covers Maintaining good medical practice, Good clinical care and Teaching and training, appraising and assessing. Sections of your portfolio to file under this domain would include most areas of CPD, audit and reflective practice, for example:

- GMC/Degree/Medical Indemnity certificates
- Educational contracts
- Foundation Achievement or equivalent
- RITA/ARCP certificates
- Learning agreements
- Personal Development Plan
- Reflective practice (for each placement)
- Examination results

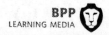

- Publications and presentations
- Audits
- Course certificates
- Mini-CEX (with summary chart if possible)
- CBD
- DOPS (with summary chart if possible)
- PBA (with summary chart if possible)
- Logbook
- Teaching attendance summary
- Self-directed teaching
- Summary of teaching delivered with feedback if possible
- Formal teaching delivered
- Extra-curricular achievements
- Evidence of specialty experience/commitment

Domain 2: Safety and quality

Put into effect systems to protect patients and improve care:

- Respond constructively to audit, involve yourself in quality assurance and improvement, comply with risk management and clinical governance procedures and provide information to assist organisations monitoring public health
- Provide adequate supervision for all staff for whom you are responsible, ensure reporting systems are in place for concerns regarding patient safety including suspected adverse drug reactions

Respond to risks to safety:

- Report risk in the healthcare environment, protect health and wellbeing of vulnerable patient groups and act if a colleague may be putting patients at risk. Comply with infection control policy and respond swiftly to risk posed by patients

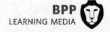

Protect patients and colleagues to any risk posed by your health:

- Have independent medical advice available to you and ensure you are immunised against serious communicable diseases for which vaccines are available

This domain covers the pillar of Health and some aspects of the pillar of Maintaining good medical practice. Sections of your portfolio to file under this domain would be as follows:

- Evidence of experience or involvement in risk management / clinical governance groups
- Reflective practice regarding issues of patient safety, risk and clinical governance
- Any audits which involve quality assurance / improvement as opposed to direct clinical issues
- Health declaration
- Health passport

Domain 3: Communication, partnership and teamwork

Communicate effectively:

- Communicate effectively with colleagues, encourage contributions from and communication between colleagues and provide information to colleagues involved in or taking over your patients' care
- Explain to patients when something has gone wrong; listen to and respect patients' views regarding their health; give them information they need to make decisions in ways they can understand; answer their questions and keep them informed; and treat those close to the patient with consideration

Work constructively with colleagues and delegate effectively:

- Treat colleagues fairly and with respect; act as a positive role model and provide effective leadership; ensure colleagues

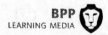

to whom you delegate have appropriate experience and support colleagues with problems

Establish and maintain partnerships with patients:

- Encourage patients to be involved with their health and decisions that affect their care, and obtain valid and informed consent before undertaking any examination, investigation, research or procedure

This domain covers aspects of the pillars of Relationships with patients and Working with colleagues. Sections of your portfolio to file under this domain would mainly include Multi-Source Feedback from both of these groups and reflective practice if appropriate.

- Self mini-PAT
- Formal colleague Multi-Source Feedback/360 degree assessments
- Informal colleague feedback (Goodbye/good luck cards)
- Formal patient feedback/360-degree assessment
- Patient informal feedback (Thank you cards)
- Reflective practice

Domain 4: Maintaining trust

Show respect for patients:

- Maintain confidentiality and support systems in place to do so, be honest, considerate and polite, treat patients with respect, as individuals and with dignity and respect the rights of patients involved in research

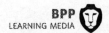

Treat patients and colleagues fairly and without discrimination:

- Be honest and impartial when assessing or appraising colleagues or providing references, and respond quickly to complaints

Act with honesty and integrity:

- Ensure you have adequate indemnity cover, be honest in all financial and commercial dealings and when writing reports or documents regarding your qualifications, experience and positions. Obtain appropriate ethical approval for research projects, be honest in performing and reporting results and ensure your research is regularly audited

This domain covers aspects of the pillars of Probity. Sections of your portfolio to file under this domain are listed below:

- Statement of probity
- CRB disclosure
- Reflective practice

To summarise, revalidation is evolving and we must be prepared to evolve how we display our evidence. However, at present it seems that annual appraisal and regular CPD will be more relevant than ever, therefore keeping a well-maintained portfolio of evidence of your competency and progression is imperative. This does not need to be much extra work, as the evidence that you require for revalidation can be drawn from your annual appraisals and the portfolio that you will already have made and updated with the pillars of Good Medical Practice in mind. Ask yourself at all times: could you demonstrate your competence in these pillars if asked to do so? If you have followed the guidance set out, the answer should be a clear yes.

Conclusion

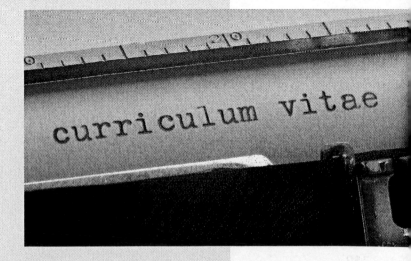

Conclusion

I hope that this guide has been useful to you, and will continue to be of use throughout your career. As mentioned, we are in a system of change, but there are certain elements of a medical career that will never alter, and overwhelming competition and the need to display evidence of your competence and suitability at every job interview, annual assessment or revalidation process are such elements. The wide variety of medical careers available at times seems overwhelming, and I would advise all of you who are in the early stages of your careers not to undertake a specialty lightly. This is the path you are choosing for potentially the next forty years, and because something seemed 'cool' at Medical School, or a relative of yours is a consultant in the specialty, does not make it suitable for you as an individual. Be guided by your instincts and regularly ask yourself if you are happy in your work. Although it is not easy to change paths once you have chosen a specialty, it is not impossible, and guidance from seniors, the BMA, MMC and the Royal Colleges is available.

Finally, remember to attend to your CV regularly to make sure it progresses as you do. It is a summary of essential information, which of course cannot possibly encapsulate you as a person or even a doctor, but it is often all the people doing the shortlisting have to go on! Do it justice and you will do yourself proud at any interview or review. Good luck.

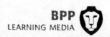

More titles in the MediPass Series

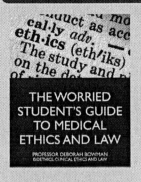

THE WORRIED STUDENT'S GUIDE TO MEDICAL ETHICS AND LAW

PROFESSOR DEBORAH BOWMAN
BIOETHICS, CLINICAL ETHICS AND LAW

£19.99

October 2011

Paperback

978-1-445379-49-4

Are you confused about medical ethics and law? Are you looking for a definitive book that will explain clearly medical ethics and law?

This book offers a unique guide to medical ethics and law for applicants to medical school, current medical students at all stages of their training, those attending postgraduate ethics courses and clinicians involved in teaching. It will also prove a useful guide for any healthcare professional with an interest in medical ethics and law. This book provides comprehensive coverage of the core curriculum (as recently revised) and clear demonstration of how to pass examinations, both written and practical. The title also considers the ethical dilemmas that students can encounter during their training.

This easy to use guide sets out to provide:

- Comprehensive coverage of the recently revised core curriculum

- Consideration of the realities of medical student experiences and dilemmas with reference to recently published and new GMC guidance for medical students

- Practical guidance on applying ethics in the clinical years, how to approach all types of examinations and improve confidence regarding the moral aspects of medicine

- A single, portable volume that covers all stages of the medical student experience

In addition to the core curriculum, this book uniquely explains the special privileges and responsibilities of being a healthcare professional and explores how professional behaviour guidance from the General Medical Council applies to students and medical professionals. The book is a single, accessible volume that will be invaluable to all those who want to thrive, not merely survive, studying and applying medical ethics day to day, whatever their stage of training.

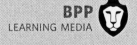

BPP
LEARNING MEDIA

More titles in the Progressing your Medical Career Series

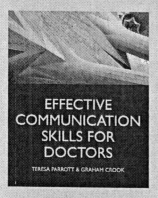

EFFECTIVE
COMMUNICATION
SKILLS FOR
DOCTORS

TERESA PARROTT & GRAHAM CROOK

£19.99

September 2011

Paperback

978-1-445379-56-2

Would you like to know how to improve your communication skills? Are you looking for a clearly written book which explores all aspects of effective medical communication?

There is an urgent need to improve doctors' communication skills. Research has shown that poor communication can contribute to patient dissatisfaction, lack of compliance and increased medico-legal problems. Improved communication skills will impact positively on all of these areas.

The last fifteen years have seen unprecedented changes in medicine and the role of doctors. Effective communication skills are vital to these new roles. But communication is not just related to personality. Skills can be learned which can make your communication more effective, and help you to improve your relationships with patients, their families and fellow doctors.

This book shows how to learn those skills and outlines why we all need to communicate more effectively. Healthcare is increasingly a partnership. Change is happening at all levels, from government directives to patient expectations. Communication is a bridge between the wisdom of the past and the vision of the future.

Readers of this book can also gain free access to an online module which upon successful completion can download a certificate for their portfolio of learning/ Revalidation/CPD records.

This easy-to-read guide will help medical students and doctors at all stages of their careers improve their communication within a hospital environment.

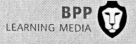

BPP
LEARNING MEDIA

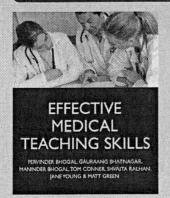
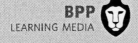

More titles in the Essential Clinical Handbook Series

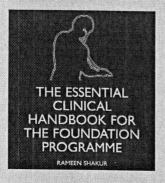

THE ESSENTIAL CLINICAL HANDBOOK FOR THE FOUNDATION PROGRAMME

RAMEEN SHAKUR

Unsure of what clinical competencies you must gain to successfully complete the Foundation Programme? Unclear on how to ensure your ePortfolio is complete to enable your progression to ST training?

This up-to-date clinical handbook is aimed at current foundation doctors and clinical medical students and provides a comprehensive companion to help you in the day-to-day management of patients on the ward. Together with this it is the first handbook to also outline clearly how to gain the core clinical competencies required for successful completion of the Foundation Programme. Written by doctors for doctors this comprehensive handbook explains how to successfully manage all of the common cases you will face during the Foundation Programme and:

- Introduces the Foundation Programme and what is expected of a new doctor especially with the introduction of Modernising Medical Careers

- Illustrates clearly the best way to manage, step-by-step, over 150 commonly encountered clinical diseases, including NICE guidelines to ensure a gold standard of clinical care is achieved.

- Describes how to successfully gain the core clinical competencies within Medicine and Surgery including an extensive list of differentials and conditions explained

- Explores the various radiology images you will encounter and how to interpret them

- Tells you how to succeed in the assessment methods used including DOP's, Mini-CEX's and CBD's.

- Has step by step diagrammatic guide to doing common clinical procedures competently and safely.

- Outlines how to ensure your ePortfolio is maintained properly to ensure successful completion of the Foundation Programme.

- Provides tips and advice on how to start preparing now to ensure you are fully prepared and have the competitive edge for your CMT/ST application.

£24.99

October 2011

Paperback

978-1-445381-63-3

The introduction of the e-Portfolio as part of the Foundation Programme has paved the way for foundation doctors to take charge of their own learning and portfolio. Through following the expert guidance laid down in this handbook you will give yourself the best possible chance of progressing successfully through to CMT/ST training.

BPP LEARNING MEDIA

www.bpp.com/health

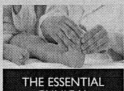
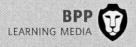

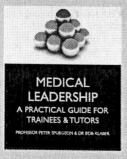
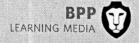